# CONTENTS

# CHAPTER 1: INTRODUCTION TO DIABETES-RELATED RETINOPATHY

## Overview of Diabetes Mellitus

Diabetes mellitus, commonly referred to as diabetes, is a chronic metabolic disorder characterized by elevated blood glucose levels, resulting from either insufficient insulin production, inadequate insulin action, or both. This condition poses a significant global health burden, affecting millions of individuals worldwide and contributing to various complications, including diabetes-related retinopathy.

## Classification of Diabetes Mellitus:

Diabetes mellitus is classified into several types, each with distinct etiologies, clinical presentations, and management strategies:

1. **Type 1 Diabetes:** This form of diabetes results from autoimmune destruction of pancreatic beta cells, leading to absolute insulin deficiency. It often manifests in childhood or early adulthood and requires lifelong insulin therapy for management.
2. **Type 2 Diabetes:** Type 2 diabetes is characterized by insulin resistance, where the body's cells become

less responsive to insulin, coupled with relative insulin deficiency. It typically develops in adulthood and is strongly associated with obesity, sedentary lifestyle, and genetic predisposition.

3. **Gestational Diabetes Mellitus (GDM):** Gestational diabetes occurs during pregnancy when hormonal changes impair insulin action, leading to elevated blood glucose levels. While it usually resolves after childbirth, it increases the risk of developing type 2 diabetes later in life for both the mother and the child.

4. **Other Specific Types:** This category includes various forms of diabetes with specific etiologies, such as genetic defects in beta cell function or insulin action, diseases of the pancreas, drug-induced diabetes, and endocrine disorders.

**Epidemiology of Diabetes Mellitus:**

The prevalence of diabetes mellitus has been steadily increasing worldwide, driven primarily by changes in lifestyle, urbanization, and an aging population. According to the International Diabetes Federation (IDF), approximately 463 million adults aged 20-79 years were living with diabetes in 2019, with projections estimating this number to rise to 700 million by 204

Type 2 diabetes accounts for the majority of diabetes cases globally, representing around 90% of all diagnoses. However, the incidence of type 1 diabetes, particularly in children, is also on the rise, indicating a complex interplay of genetic and environmental factors in disease development.

Certain populations, such as indigenous peoples, ethnic minorities, and socioeconomically disadvantaged groups, are disproportionately affected by diabetes, highlighting the importance of addressing health disparities and implementing culturally sensitive interventions.

## Pathophysiology of Diabetes Mellitus:

The pathophysiology of diabetes mellitus involves intricate mechanisms that disrupt glucose homeostasis, leading to hyperglycemia and subsequent tissue damage. In type 1 diabetes, autoimmune destruction of pancreatic beta cells results in an absolute deficiency of insulin, impairing glucose uptake by peripheral tissues and promoting hepatic glucose production. Conversely, type 2 diabetes is characterized by insulin resistance, where adipose tissue, skeletal muscle, and liver cells exhibit reduced responsiveness to insulin signaling, leading to compensatory hyperinsulinemia and eventual beta cell failure.

Chronic hyperglycemia contributes to the development of microvascular and macrovascular complications, including diabetic retinopathy, nephropathy, neuropathy, cardiovascular disease, and stroke. Additionally, dysregulated lipid metabolism, inflammation, oxidative stress, and endothelial dysfunction play crucial roles in the pathogenesis of diabetic complications, exacerbating tissue damage and impairing organ function.

In conclusion, diabetes mellitus is a complex metabolic disorder characterized by dysregulated glucose metabolism, with type 1 and type 2 diabetes representing the most common forms of the disease. Its increasing prevalence poses significant challenges to global public health, necessitating comprehensive strategies for prevention, early detection, and management. Understanding the pathophysiology and epidemiology of diabetes mellitus is essential for developing targeted interventions to mitigate its impact on individuals and society as a whole.

## Definition and Classification of Diabetic Retinopathy

Diabetic retinopathy (DR) is a potentially sight-threatening complication of diabetes mellitus, characterized by progressive damage to the microvasculature of the retina. It is one of the leading causes of blindness among working-age adults worldwide, highlighting the critical importance of early detection, timely intervention, and effective management strategies.

## Classification of Diabetic Retinopathy:

Diabetic retinopathy encompasses a spectrum of pathological changes that evolve over time, ranging from mild non-proliferative changes to severe proliferative disease with vision-threatening complications. Understanding the classification system is essential for accurate diagnosis, prognostication, and treatment planning. The classification of diabetic retinopathy is primarily based on clinical findings observed during ophthalmic examination, including fundoscopy, optical coherence tomography (OCT), and fluorescein angiography.

1. **Non-Proliferative Diabetic Retinopathy (NPDR):** Non-proliferative diabetic retinopathy is the early stage of the disease characterized by microvascular abnormalities, including retinal hemorrhages, microaneurysms, intraretinal microvascular abnormalities (IRMAs), venous beading, and cotton-wool spots. These changes reflect the progressive damage to retinal capillaries and the breakdown of the blood-retinal barrier due to chronic hyperglycemia. NPDR is further classified into mild, moderate, and severe stages based on the severity and extent of retinal lesions observed on fundoscopic examination.

2. **Proliferative Diabetic Retinopathy (PDR):** Proliferative diabetic retinopathy represents the advanced stage of the disease characterized by the growth of abnormal new blood vessels (neovascularization) on the surface of the

retina or optic disc. These fragile vessels are prone to leakage, leading to vitreous hemorrhage, fibrosis, and tractional retinal detachment, all of which can cause severe visual impairment or blindness if left untreated. PDR is associated with ischemia-induced angiogenic factors, such as vascular endothelial growth factor (VEGF), which promote the formation of new blood vessels in response to retinal hypoxia.

3. **Diabetic Macular Edema (DME):** Diabetic macular edema is a common complication of both NPDR and PDR, characterized by the accumulation of fluid within the macula, the central part of the retina responsible for sharp, central vision. DME occurs due to increased vascular permeability and breakdown of the blood-retinal barrier, leading to fluid leakage from retinal capillaries into the surrounding tissue. It is a significant cause of visual impairment in patients with diabetic retinopathy and requires prompt intervention to prevent irreversible vision loss.

## Risk Factors for Diabetic Retinopathy:

Several factors contribute to the development and progression of diabetic retinopathy, including:

- Duration of diabetes: The risk of developing diabetic retinopathy increases with the duration of diabetes, with longer disease duration correlating with a higher prevalence and severity of retinal lesions.
- Glycemic control: Poorly controlled diabetes, characterized by persistent hyperglycemia and glycemic variability, accelerates the onset and progression of diabetic retinopathy by promoting microvascular damage and retinal ischemia.
- Hypertension: Systemic hypertension is a significant risk factor for diabetic retinopathy, as it exacerbates retinal vascular dysfunction and increases the likelihood of

developing macular edema and retinal ischemia.

- Hyperlipidemia: Dyslipidemia, characterized by elevated levels of triglycerides, low-density lipoprotein (LDL) cholesterol, and decreased high-density lipoprotein (HDL) cholesterol, is associated with an increased risk of diabetic retinopathy and progression to advanced stages of the disease.
- Genetic predisposition: Genetic factors play a role in the pathogenesis of diabetic retinopathy, with certain genetic polymorphisms predisposing individuals to a higher risk of developing retinal microvascular complications in the setting of diabetes mellitus.

In conclusion, diabetic retinopathy is a sight-threatening complication of diabetes mellitus characterized by progressive damage to the microvasculature of the retina. The classification system distinguishes between non-proliferative and proliferative stages of the disease, each with distinct clinical features, prognoses, and management approaches. Early detection, regular screening, and optimal management of modifiable risk factors are essential for preventing or delaying the onset and progression of diabetic retinopathy and preserving visual function in affected individuals.

## Epidemiology and Risk Factors of Diabetic Retinopathy

Diabetic retinopathy (DR) is a prevalent microvascular complication of diabetes mellitus, affecting a substantial proportion of individuals with both type 1 and type 2 diabetes worldwide. Understanding the epidemiology and risk factors associated with DR is essential for implementing effective preventive strategies, early detection programs, and targeted interventions to mitigate its impact on visual health and overall well-being.

**Epidemiology of Diabetic Retinopathy:**

The epidemiology of diabetic retinopathy varies across different populations, influenced by factors such as the prevalence of diabetes, demographic characteristics, access to healthcare services, and quality of diabetes management. However, several key epidemiological trends are observed globally:

1. **Prevalence**: Diabetic retinopathy is one of the most common complications of diabetes mellitus, affecting approximately one-third of individuals with diabetes worldwide. The prevalence of DR increases with the duration of diabetes, with estimates suggesting that up to 80% of patients with diabetes for 20 years or more will develop some degree of retinopathy.

2. **Type of Diabetes**: While both type 1 and type 2 diabetes are associated with the development of diabetic retinopathy, the prevalence and severity of DR differ between the two types. Historically, type 1 diabetes was considered to have a higher risk of retinopathy due to earlier onset and longer disease duration. However, with the rising prevalence of type 2 diabetes, particularly in younger age groups, the burden of DR in individuals with type 2 diabetes has become increasingly significant.

3. **Geographical Variation**: The prevalence of diabetic retinopathy varies geographically, with higher rates observed in regions with a higher prevalence of diabetes, such as North America, Europe, and parts of Asia. However, diabetic retinopathy is also a significant public health concern in low- and middle-income countries, where access to screening and treatment services may be limited, leading to higher rates of vision-threatening complications.

4. **Impact on Visual Health**: Diabetic retinopathy is a leading

cause of visual impairment and blindness among working-age adults globally. Vision-threatening complications, such as diabetic macular edema (DME), proliferative diabetic retinopathy (PDR), and vitreous hemorrhage, can significantly impact an individual's quality of life and socioeconomic productivity if left untreated.

**Risk Factors for Diabetic Retinopathy:**

Several risk factors contribute to the development and progression of diabetic retinopathy, including:

1. **Duration of Diabetes**: The risk of developing diabetic retinopathy increases with the duration of diabetes, with longer disease duration associated with a higher prevalence and severity of retinal microvascular complications. This relationship underscores the importance of early detection and regular screening for diabetic retinopathy in individuals with diabetes, particularly those with longstanding disease.

2. **Glycemic Control**: Chronic hyperglycemia is a major risk factor for the development and progression of diabetic retinopathy. Prolonged exposure to elevated blood glucose levels promotes microvascular damage, endothelial dysfunction, and retinal ischemia, contributing to the pathogenesis of retinopathy. Intensive glycemic control through lifestyle modifications, antidiabetic medications, and insulin therapy has been shown to reduce the risk of diabetic retinopathy and slow its progression in patients with diabetes.

3. **Hypertension**: Systemic hypertension is a significant risk factor for diabetic retinopathy, as it exacerbates retinal vascular dysfunction and promotes the development of microvascular complications. Hypertension-induced arteriolar narrowing, endothelial damage, and increased vascular permeability contribute to retinal ischemia,

neovascularization, and macular edema in patients with diabetes. Optimal blood pressure control, through lifestyle modifications and antihypertensive medications, is essential for preventing and managing diabetic retinopathy in hypertensive individuals.

4. **Dyslipidemia**: Dyslipidemia, characterized by elevated levels of triglycerides, low-density lipoprotein (LDL) cholesterol, and decreased high-density lipoprotein (HDL) cholesterol, is associated with an increased risk of diabetic retinopathy and progression to advanced stages of the disease. Dyslipidemia promotes atherosclerosis, endothelial dysfunction, and microvascular damage, exacerbating retinal ischemia and neovascularization in patients with diabetes. Lipid-lowering therapies, such as statins and fibrates, may reduce the risk of diabetic retinopathy and improve visual outcomes in individuals with dyslipidemia and diabetes.

5. **Genetic Predisposition**: Genetic factors play a significant role in the pathogenesis of diabetic retinopathy, with certain genetic polymorphisms predisposing individuals to a higher risk of developing retinal microvascular complications in the setting of diabetes mellitus. Genome-wide association studies (GWAS) have identified several susceptibility loci associated with diabetic retinopathy, including genes involved in angiogenesis, inflammation, oxidative stress, and lipid metabolism. Understanding the genetic basis of diabetic retinopathy may facilitate risk stratification, early detection, and personalized management approaches in patients with diabetes.

6. **Other Risk Factors**: Additional risk factors for diabetic retinopathy include smoking, pregnancy, nephropathy, pregnancy, and pregnancy-induced hypertension. Smoking is a modifiable risk factor that exacerbates microvascular damage, oxidative stress, and inflammation in patients with diabetes, increasing the risk of

retinopathy and other diabetic complications. Pregnancy and pregnancy-induced hypertension are associated with transient worsening of diabetic retinopathy due to hormonal changes, increased metabolic demands, and hemodynamic alterations during pregnancy. Diabetic nephropathy, characterized by proteinuria and declining renal function, is a significant risk factor for the development and progression of diabetic retinopathy, reflecting systemic microvascular dysfunction and endothelial damage in patients with diabetes.

In conclusion, diabetic retinopathy is a prevalent microvascular complication of diabetes mellitus, affecting a substantial proportion of individuals with both type 1 and type 2 diabetes worldwide. The epidemiology of diabetic retinopathy varies across different populations, influenced by factors such as the prevalence of diabetes, demographic characteristics, access to healthcare services, and quality of diabetes management. Several risk factors contribute to the development and progression of diabetic retinopathy, including the duration of diabetes, glycemic control, hypertension, dyslipidemia, genetic predisposition, smoking, pregnancy, and nephropathy. Understanding these risk factors is essential for implementing effective preventive strategies, early detection programs, and targeted interventions to mitigate the impact of diabetic retinopathy on visual health and overall well-being.

## Pathophysiology of Diabetes-Related Retinopathy

Diabetes-related retinopathy (DR) is a complex and multifactorial microvascular complication of diabetes mellitus that affects the retina, the light-sensitive tissue lining the inner surface of the eye. The pathophysiology of DR involves a cascade of interconnected molecular, cellular, and structural changes within the retinal microvasculature, driven primarily by chronic hyperglycemia and metabolic dysregulation. Understanding the underlying pathophysiological mechanisms is crucial for elucidating the disease process, identifying therapeutic targets, and developing effective interventions to prevent or mitigate the progression of DR.

### Chronic Hyperglycemia and Metabolic Dysregulation:

Chronic hyperglycemia is the hallmark feature of diabetes mellitus and plays a central role in the pathogenesis of DR. Prolonged exposure to elevated glucose levels leads to metabolic dysregulation and cellular dysfunction in various retinal cell types, including endothelial cells, pericytes, Müller cells, astrocytes, and neurons.

1. **Endothelial Dysfunction:** Hyperglycemia-induced endothelial dysfunction is a key initiating event in the development of DR. Endothelial cells lining the retinal microvasculature become activated and dysfunctional in response to high glucose levels, leading to impaired vasodilation, increased vascular permeability, and abnormal angiogenic signaling. Dysfunctional endothelial cells contribute to the breakdown of the blood-retinal barrier (BRB), facilitating the leakage of plasma proteins and inflammatory mediators into the surrounding retinal tissue.

2. **Pericyte Loss and Capillary Basement Membrane Thickening:** Pericytes are specialized contractile cells that ensheath retinal capillaries and regulate microvascular tone and permeability. Chronic hyperglycemia induces pericyte apoptosis and loss, resulting in capillary dropout and microaneurysm formation. Additionally, thickening of the capillary basement membrane, secondary to increased deposition of extracellular matrix proteins

such as collagen and fibronectin, contributes to vascular occlusion and ischemia in the diabetic retina.

3. **Müller Cell Activation and Neuroglial Dysfunction:** Müller cells are the principal glial cells of the retina and play a crucial role in maintaining retinal homeostasis and supporting neuronal function. In response to hyperglycemia and oxidative stress, Müller cells undergo reactive gliosis, characterized by cellular hypertrophy, proliferation, and upregulation of pro-inflammatory cytokines and growth factors. Activated Müller cells contribute to neuroglial dysfunction, synaptic remodeling, and neuronal apoptosis in the diabetic retina, exacerbating retinal neurodegeneration and functional impairment.

4. **Oxidative Stress and Inflammatory Mediators:** Chronic hyperglycemia promotes the generation of reactive oxygen species (ROS) and oxidative stress in the diabetic retina, leading to lipid peroxidation, protein oxidation, and DNA damage. Oxidative stress activates various pro-inflammatory signaling pathways, including nuclear factor-kappa B (NF-κB) and mitogen-activated protein kinases (MAPKs), resulting in the production of inflammatory mediators such as cytokines, chemokines, adhesion molecules, and prostaglandins. Inflammatory mediators contribute to leukocyte recruitment, microglial activation, and amplification of retinal inflammation, exacerbating tissue damage and neurovascular dysfunction in DR.

**Angiogenic and Vasoactive Factors:**

Dysregulated expression of angiogenic and vasoactive factors plays a critical role in the progression of DR, leading to aberrant neovascularization, vascular leakage, and retinal ischemia. Several key factors implicated in DR pathophysiology include:

1. **Vascular Endothelial Growth Factor (VEGF):** VEGF is a potent angiogenic factor that stimulates endothelial cell proliferation, migration, and vascular permeability. In the diabetic retina, upregulation of VEGF expression in response to hypoxia and oxidative stress promotes the growth of abnormal new blood vessels (neovascularization) on the surface of the retina or optic disc, contributing to proliferative diabetic retinopathy (PDR) and diabetic macular edema (DME).

2. **Insulin-like Growth Factor-1 (IGF-1):** IGF-1 is a growth-promoting peptide that regulates cell proliferation, survival, and differentiation. Elevated levels of IGF-1 in the diabetic retina promote angiogenesis, fibrosis, and neuroglial dysfunction, exacerbating the progression of DR. IGF-1 signaling interacts synergistically with VEGF and other growth factors to promote pathological neovascularization and vascular leakage in the diabetic retina.

3. **Platelet-Derived Growth Factor (PDGF):** PDGF is a potent mitogen and chemoattractant that regulates the proliferation and migration of pericytes, smooth muscle cells, and fibroblasts. Dysregulated PDGF signaling in the diabetic retina contributes to pericyte loss, capillary dropout, and vascular remodeling, exacerbating microvascular dysfunction and ischemia in DR.

4. **Endothelin-1 (ET-1):** ET-1 is a vasoconstrictor peptide produced by endothelial cells and pericytes that regulates vascular tone and permeability. Elevated levels of ET-1 in the diabetic retina promote vasoconstriction, vascular remodeling, and inflammation, contributing to retinal ischemia and neovascularization in DR. ET-1 antagonists have shown promise as potential therapeutic agents for the treatment of DR by mitigating microvascular dysfunction and neurovascular coupling in the diabetic retina.

## Neurovascular Crosstalk and Retinal Remodeling:

The pathophysiology of DR involves complex interactions between vascular and neuronal elements of the retina, leading to neurovascular uncoupling, synaptic dysfunction, and retinal remodeling. Chronic hyperglycemia and oxidative stress induce neuroglial dysfunction, synaptic remodeling, and neuronal apoptosis in the diabetic retina, contributing to visual impairment and functional deficits in DR. Conversely, retinal neurodegeneration and neuroinflammation exacerbate microvascular dysfunction and tissue damage, creating a feedforward cycle of neurovascular crosstalk and pathological remodeling in the diabetic retina.

In conclusion, the pathophysiology of diabetes-related retinopathy is characterized by a cascade of interconnected molecular, cellular, and structural changes within the retinal microvasculature, driven primarily by chronic hyperglycemia, metabolic dysregulation, and dysregulated expression of angiogenic and vasoactive factors. Endothelial dysfunction, pericyte loss, Müller cell activation, oxidative stress, and inflammatory mediators contribute to microvascular damage, neuroglial dysfunction, and retinal neurodegeneration in DR. Angiogenic and vasoactive factors such as VEGF, IGF-1, PDGF, and ET-1 play critical roles in promoting pathological neovascularization, vascular leakage, and retinal ischemia in DR. Neurovascular crosstalk and retinal remodeling further exacerbate tissue damage and functional impairment in the diabetic retina, highlighting the complexity of DR pathophysiology and the need for targeted therapeutic interventions to preserve visual function and prevent vision loss in affected individuals.

# CHAPTER 2: ANATOMY AND PHYSIOLOGY OF THE RETINA

**Structure of the Retina**

The retina is a highly specialized neural tissue located in the posterior segment of the eye, lining the inner surface of the eyeball. It plays a crucial role in vision by capturing and processing light signals and transmitting visual information to the brain via the optic nerve. The retina consists of several distinct layers, each containing specialized cells and structures that contribute to its function. Understanding the anatomy and organization of the retina is essential for comprehending its role in visual perception and the pathophysiology of retinal diseases, including diabetic retinopathy.

**Layers of the Retina:**

The retina is composed of ten histologically distinct layers, arranged in a laminar fashion from the outermost layer adjacent to the choroid to the innermost layer facing the vitreous humor. These layers can be broadly categorized into three main regions: the photoreceptor layer, the inner nuclear layer, and the ganglion cell layer.

1. **Photoreceptor Layer:**
   - **Outer Segment:** The outer segment of photoreceptor cells contains specialized structures called photoreceptor discs, which house the photopigments responsible for capturing light signals. In humans, there are two types of photoreceptors: rods and cones. Rods are responsible for low-light vision and peripheral vision, while cones are responsible for color vision and high-acuity vision.
   - **Inner Segment:** The inner segment contains the cell's nucleus and various organelles involved in protein synthesis and energy metabolism.
   - **Synaptic Terminal:** The synaptic terminal forms connections with bipolar cells, transmitting visual signals from photoreceptors to downstream retinal neurons.
2. **Inner Nuclear Layer:**
   - **Bipolar Cells:** Bipolar cells receive input from photoreceptor cells and transmit visual signals to ganglion cells. There are several subtypes of bipolar cells, each with distinct anatomical and functional properties.
   - **Horizontal Cells:** Horizontal cells modulate the activity of photoreceptors and bipolar cells, contributing to lateral inhibition and contrast enhancement in visual processing.
   - **Amacrine Cells:** Amacrine cells integrate and modulate visual signals within the inner nuclear layer, mediating interactions between bipolar cells and ganglion cells and contributing to motion detection and spatial filtering.
3. **Ganglion Cell Layer:**

- **Ganglion Cells:** Ganglion cells are the output neurons of the retina, transmitting visual signals to the brain via the optic nerve. They receive input from bipolar cells and amacrine cells and integrate this information to generate action potentials that propagate along their axons.
- **Ganglion Cell Axons:** Ganglion cell axons converge at the optic disc, forming the optic nerve, which carries visual information from the retina to the brain for further processing.

In addition to these primary layers, the retina also contains several supporting cell types and structures that contribute to its function and integrity:

- **Müller Cells:** Müller cells are radial glial cells that span the entire thickness of the retina, providing structural support, metabolic maintenance, and neurotransmitter recycling. They also contribute to the maintenance of the blood-retinal barrier and play a role in regulating extracellular ion and water homeostasis.
- **Retinal Pigment Epithelium (RPE):** The RPE is a single layer of pigmented cells located adjacent to the photoreceptor layer, between the retina and the choroid. It functions to nourish and support the photoreceptor cells, absorb excess light, recycle visual pigments, and maintain the integrity of the outer blood-retinal barrier.
- **Choroid:** The choroid is a highly vascularized layer located between the retina and the sclera, providing oxygen and nutrients to the outer layers of the retina. It also helps regulate the temperature and hydration of the retina and absorbs excess light to prevent glare and improve visual acuity.

**Microarchitecture of the Retina:**

The microarchitecture of the retina exhibits regional variations in cellular density, synaptic connectivity, and functional specialization, reflecting its role in processing visual information across different regions of the visual field. The fovea, located at the center of the macula, contains a high density of cone photoreceptors and ganglion cells, providing high-acuity vision and color discrimination. Surrounding the fovea is the parafoveal region, which contains a mixture of cones and rods and contributes to peripheral vision and motion detection. The peripheral retina, located outside the macula, contains predominantly rods and contributes to low-light vision and spatial awareness.

**Blood Supply and Vasculature:**

The retina receives its blood supply from two distinct vascular systems: the central retinal artery and the choroidal circulation. The central retinal artery enters the eye through the optic nerve head and branches into arterioles that supply the inner layers of the retina, including the ganglion cell layer and the inner nuclear layer. The choroidal circulation, located in the choroid, supplies oxygen and nutrients to the outer layers of the retina, including the photoreceptor layer and the retinal pigment epithelium. The retinal vasculature is organized into distinct layers, including the superficial retinal vessels, the deep retinal capillary plexus, and the intermediate and deep vascular plexuses, each serving specific regions of the retina and contributing to its metabolic and functional demands.

In summary, the retina is a complex and highly organized neural tissue that plays a critical role in vision by capturing, processing, and transmitting visual information to the brain. Its layered structure consists of specialized cell types and structures that contribute to its function and integrity, including photoreceptors, bipolar cells, ganglion cells, Müller cells, and the retinal pigment epithelium. The microarchitecture of the retina exhibits regional variations in cellular density and synaptic connectivity, reflecting its role in processing visual information across different regions of the visual field. Understanding the structure and organization of the retina is essential for comprehending its role in visual perception and the pathophysiology of retinal diseases, including diabetic retinopathy.

## Function of the Retina

The retina is a highly specialized neural tissue located at the back of the eye, lining the inner surface of the eyeball. Its primary function is to capture, process, and transmit visual information to the brain, enabling the perception of light, shapes, colors, and motion. The retina accomplishes these complex tasks through the coordinated activity of its various cell types and layers, each contributing to specific aspects of visual processing. Understanding the function of the retina is essential for comprehending the mechanisms underlying visual perception and the pathophysiology of retinal diseases, including diabetic retinopathy.

## Visual Transduction:

At the core of retinal function lies the process of visual transduction, whereby light signals are converted into electrical signals that can be interpreted by the brain. This process occurs within the photoreceptor cells, specialized sensory neurons located in the outermost layer of the retina. Photoreceptors contain light-sensitive pigments called photopigments, which undergo a series of conformational changes in response to light exposure. In humans, there are two main types of photoreceptors: rods and cones.

- **Rods:** Rod photoreceptors are highly sensitive to dim light and are responsible for scotopic (low-light) vision. They contain the photopigment rhodopsin, which absorbs light in the blue-green spectrum. Rods are abundant in the peripheral retina and play a crucial role in night vision and peripheral vision.
- **Cones:** Cone photoreceptors are responsible for photopic (daylight) vision and color perception. There are three subtypes of cones, each containing a different photopigment that absorbs light in either the short-wavelength (blue), medium-wavelength (green), or long-wavelength (red) part of the spectrum. Cones are concentrated in the central region of the retina, particularly in the fovea, where visual acuity is highest.

When light strikes the photoreceptor outer segments, it triggers a cascade of biochemical reactions that lead to the hyperpolarization of the photoreceptor cell membrane. This hyperpolarization generates a neural signal that is transmitted to downstream retinal neurons for further processing.

**Signal Processing:**

Visual signals captured by photoreceptors are transmitted to bipolar cells, interneurons located in the inner nuclear layer of the retina. Bipolar cells receive input from multiple photoreceptors and integrate this information to generate spatial and temporal patterns of neural activity. There are two main types of bipolar cells: ON-center bipolar cells and OFF-center bipolar cells.

- **ON-center Bipolar Cells:** ON-center bipolar cells depolarize in response to increases in light intensity, signifying the presence of a light stimulus in their receptive field center. They receive excitatory input from cones and rods via synapses in the outer plexiform layer.
- **OFF-center Bipolar Cells:** OFF-center bipolar cells depolarize in response to decreases in light intensity,

signifying the absence of a light stimulus in their receptive field center. They receive inhibitory input from cones and rods via synapses in the outer plexiform layer.

Bipolar cells transmit visual signals to ganglion cells, the output neurons of the retina located in the ganglion cell layer. Ganglion cells integrate input from bipolar cells and other retinal interneurons and generate action potentials in response to specific patterns of light stimulation. There are several subtypes of ganglion cells, each with distinct anatomical and functional properties, including receptive field size, spatial resolution, and sensitivity to motion and contrast.

**Transmission to the Brain:**

Axons of ganglion cells converge at the optic disc, forming the optic nerve, which carries visual information from the retina to the brain for further processing. The optic nerve fibers from each eye converge at the optic chiasm, where they undergo partial decussation, with fibers from the nasal retina crossing to the contralateral hemisphere and fibers from the temporal retina remaining ipsilateral. Visual information is then relayed to various visual processing centers in the brain, including the lateral geniculate nucleus (LGN) of the thalamus, the primary visual cortex (V1) in the occipital lobe, and higher-order visual areas responsible for object recognition, motion perception, and visual memory.

**Non-Image-Forming Functions:**

In addition to its role in conscious vision, the retina also contributes to various non-image-forming functions, including circadian rhythm regulation, pupillary light reflex, and modulation of refractive development. Specialized retinal ganglion cells, known as intrinsically photosensitive retinal ganglion cells (ipRGCs), contain the photopigment melanopsin and are sensitive to light signals that regulate these non-image-forming functions. ipRGCs project to the suprachiasmatic nucleus (SCN) of the hypothalamus, the master circadian pacemaker, and other brain regions involved in autonomic control and behavioral responses to light.

In summary, the retina plays a central role in vision by capturing, processing, and transmitting visual information to the brain. Photoreceptors detect light signals and initiate the process of visual transduction, converting light energy into electrical signals that are transmitted to bipolar cells. Bipolar cells integrate and modulate visual signals before transmitting them to ganglion cells, which generate action potentials and convey visual information to the brain via the optic nerve. The retina also contributes to various non-image-forming functions, including circadian rhythm regulation and pupillary light reflex, through specialized retinal ganglion cells. Understanding the function of the retina is essential for comprehending visual perception and the mechanisms underlying retinal diseases, including diabetic retinopathy, and developing targeted therapeutic interventions to preserve visual function and improve quality of life.

## Blood Supply to the Retina

The retina, a highly metabolically active tissue responsible for visual perception, receives its blood supply from two distinct vascular systems: the central retinal artery and the choroidal circulation. This dual blood supply ensures adequate oxygenation and nutrient delivery to the various layers of the retina, supporting its physiological functions and maintaining tissue integrity. Understanding the anatomy and physiology of the retinal vasculature is essential for comprehending the pathophysiology of retinal diseases, including diabetic retinopathy, and developing targeted therapeutic strategies to preserve visual function.

## Anatomy of the Retinal Vasculature:

The retinal vasculature consists of a complex network of arteries, arterioles, capillaries, venules, and veins that supply blood to the inner layers of the retina. The central retinal artery, a branch of the ophthalmic artery, enters the eye through the optic nerve head and travels along the nerve fiber layer to reach the inner retinal layers. The central retinal artery then branches into arterioles that supply oxygenated blood to the retinal ganglion cells, inner nuclear layer, and inner plexiform layer. Arterioles further divide into a dense network of capillaries, forming the superficial and deep retinal capillary plexuses that nourish the inner retinal layers.

In addition to the central retinal artery, the retina also receives blood supply from the choroidal circulation, a network of blood vessels located in the choroid, a vascular layer between the retina and the sclera. Choroidal vessels supply oxygenated blood to the outer layers of the retina, including the photoreceptor layer and the retinal pigment epithelium (RPE). Choroidal arteries penetrate the sclera and branch into arterioles that supply the choriocapillaris, a highly fenestrated capillary network adjacent to the RPE. Capillaries of the choriocapillaris form an intricate meshwork that provides oxygen and nutrients to the photoreceptor outer segments and removes metabolic waste products.

## Physiology of Retinal Blood Flow:

The regulation of retinal blood flow is a dynamic process governed by various physiological factors, including metabolic demand, neural activity, autoregulation, and neurovascular coupling. Blood flow to the retina must be tightly regulated to meet the metabolic demands of retinal neurons and maintain tissue homeostasis under changing physiological conditions. Several mechanisms contribute to the autoregulation of retinal blood flow:

1. **Myogenic Mechanism:** Changes in arterial pressure and vascular tone within the retinal arterioles regulate blood flow by altering vascular resistance. Increased arterial pressure leads to vasoconstriction of retinal arterioles, whereas decreased pressure results in vasodilation, ensuring stable blood flow to the retina despite fluctuations in systemic blood pressure.

2. **Metabolic Mechanism:** Local metabolic factors, such as oxygen tension, carbon dioxide levels, and pH, regulate retinal blood flow in response to changes in metabolic demand. Increased neuronal activity and metabolic demand in the retina lead to the release of vasodilatory factors, such as adenosine and nitric oxide, which promote arteriolar vasodilation and enhance blood flow to active regions of the retina.

3. **Neurovascular Coupling:** Neuronal activity in the retina, particularly in response to visual stimulation, is coupled to changes in local blood flow through neurovascular coupling mechanisms. Active neurons release neurotransmitters and neuromodulators that dilate nearby arterioles, increasing blood flow to regions of heightened neural activity. This neurovascular coupling ensures a rapid and localized response to visual stimuli, facilitating visual processing and perception.

## Clinical Implications:

Disruption of retinal blood flow regulation and vascular dysfunction play critical roles in the pathogenesis of various retinal diseases, including diabetic retinopathy, retinal vein occlusion, and age-related macular degeneration. In diabetic retinopathy, chronic hyperglycemia and metabolic dysregulation lead to microvascular damage, endothelial dysfunction, and impaired autoregulation of retinal blood flow. These changes result in capillary dropout, ischemia, and neovascularization, contributing to vision-threatening complications such as diabetic macular edema and proliferative diabetic retinopathy.

Evaluation of retinal blood flow and vascular function is essential for the diagnosis, monitoring, and management of retinal diseases. Non-invasive imaging techniques, such as fluorescein angiography, optical coherence tomography angiography (OCTA), and Doppler ultrasonography, allow clinicians to assess retinal perfusion, vascular morphology, and blood flow dynamics in vivo. These imaging modalities provide valuable information about the severity and progression of retinal vascular diseases, guiding treatment decisions and monitoring therapeutic responses.

Therapeutic strategies aimed at preserving retinal blood flow and improving vascular function are crucial for preventing or delaying the onset and progression of retinal diseases. Pharmacological agents targeting vasodilation, endothelial function, and inflammation may help restore retinal perfusion and mitigate vascular dysfunction in patients with diabetic retinopathy and other retinal disorders. Additionally, lifestyle modifications, such as optimizing glycemic control, managing systemic hypertension, and promoting healthy lifestyle habits, may improve retinal vascular health and reduce the risk of vision loss in at-risk individuals.

In summary, the retina receives its blood supply from two distinct vascular systems: the central retinal artery and the choroidal circulation. The regulation of retinal blood flow is governed by various physiological mechanisms, including myogenic, metabolic, and neurovascular coupling mechanisms, which ensure adequate oxygenation and nutrient delivery to retinal tissues under changing physiological conditions. Disruption of retinal blood flow regulation and vascular function contributes to the pathogenesis of retinal diseases, highlighting the importance of evaluating and managing retinal vascular health in clinical practice.

# CHAPTER 3: BIOCHEMICAL PATHWAYS IMPLICATED IN DIABETIC RETINOPATHY

## Hyperglycemia and its Effects on Retinal Tissue

Hyperglycemia, a hallmark feature of diabetes mellitus, exerts profound and multifaceted effects on retinal tissue, contributing to the pathogenesis of diabetic retinopathy (DR), a leading cause of vision loss and blindness worldwide. Chronic exposure to elevated blood glucose levels induces a cascade of molecular, cellular, and structural changes within the retina, leading to vascular dysfunction, neurodegeneration, and inflammatory responses. Understanding the mechanisms underlying the effects of hyperglycemia on retinal tissue is essential for elucidating the pathophysiology of DR and developing targeted therapeutic interventions to prevent or mitigate its progression.

**Molecular and Cellular Mechanisms:**

1. **Increased Formation of Advanced Glycation End Products (AGEs):** Hyperglycemia promotes the non-enzymatic glycation of proteins and lipids, leading to the formation of advanced glycation end products (AGEs) within retinal tissues. AGEs contribute to retinal damage by inducing oxidative stress, inflammation, and endothelial dysfunction, exacerbating microvascular complications in DR.

2. **Activation of Protein Kinase C (PKC) Pathway:** Hyperglycemia activates the protein kinase C (PKC) pathway in retinal cells, leading to increased vascular permeability, aberrant angiogenesis, and leukocyte adhesion. PKC-mediated signaling cascades contribute to the development of retinal microvascular abnormalities, such as capillary leakage, microaneurysm formation, and neovascularization, characteristic of DR.

3. **Oxidative Stress and Mitochondrial Dysfunction:** Chronic hyperglycemia induces oxidative stress and mitochondrial dysfunction in retinal cells, leading to increased production of reactive oxygen species (ROS) and impaired antioxidant defense mechanisms. Oxidative stress contributes to retinal damage by promoting lipid peroxidation, protein oxidation, DNA damage, and apoptosis, exacerbating neurovascular dysfunction in DR.

4. **Activation of Inflammatory Pathways:** Hyperglycemia triggers the activation of inflammatory pathways in retinal tissues, leading to the production of pro-inflammatory cytokines, chemokines, and adhesion molecules. Inflammatory mediators promote leukocyte infiltration, microglial activation, and endothelial dysfunction, contributing to retinal neuroinflammation and vascular damage in DR.

## Vascular Dysfunction and Microvascular Complications:

1. **Breakdown of Blood-Retinal Barrier (BRB):** Chronic hyperglycemia disrupts the integrity of the blood-retinal barrier (BRB), a specialized barrier formed by tight junctions between retinal endothelial cells and the retinal pigment epithelium (RPE). Increased permeability of the BRB leads to leakage of plasma proteins, inflammatory mediators, and fluid into the retinal tissue, contributing to macular edema and retinal hemorrhage in DR.

2. **Capillary Non-Perfusion and Ischemia:** Hyperglycemia induces capillary dropout and retinal ischemia through mechanisms such as pericyte loss, endothelial cell apoptosis, and microvascular occlusion. Capillary non-perfusion disrupts retinal perfusion and oxygen delivery, leading to tissue hypoxia, upregulation of angiogenic factors, and neovascularization in advanced stages of DR.

3. **Development of Microaneurysms and Hemorrhages:** Chronic hyperglycemia promotes the formation of microaneurysms, dilated capillary outpouchings that are vulnerable to rupture and hemorrhage. Microaneurysms and retinal hemorrhages contribute to vascular leakage, macular edema, and retinal fibrosis, further compromising visual function and retinal integrity in DR.

## Neurodegeneration and Functional Impairment:

1. **Loss of Retinal Neurons:** Hyperglycemia induces neurodegeneration in the retina by promoting apoptosis of retinal neurons, including ganglion cells, amacrine cells, and photoreceptors. Neuronal loss contributes to functional deficits in visual processing, contrast sensitivity, and color vision, impairing visual acuity and quality of life in individuals with DR.

2. **Impaired Neurovascular Coupling:** Hyperglycemia

disrupts neurovascular coupling mechanisms in the retina, impairing the dynamic regulation of blood flow in response to neuronal activity. Dysfunctional neurovascular coupling leads to mismatched oxygen supply and demand, exacerbating retinal hypoxia, oxidative stress, and neuroinflammation in DR.

3. **Altered Synaptic Transmission:** Hyperglycemia alters synaptic transmission and neurotransmitter release in the retina, impairing signal processing and synaptic plasticity in retinal circuits. Dysregulated synaptic transmission contributes to functional deficits in visual information processing, motion detection, and spatial orientation, exacerbating visual impairment in DR.

**Therapeutic Implications:**

Understanding the effects of hyperglycemia on retinal tissue is crucial for developing targeted therapeutic interventions to prevent or mitigate the progression of DR. Pharmacological agents targeting molecular pathways involved in oxidative stress, inflammation, and vascular dysfunction may help preserve retinal function and prevent vision loss in individuals with diabetes. Additionally, lifestyle modifications, such as optimizing glycemic control, managing systemic hypertension, and promoting healthy lifestyle habits, may reduce the risk of retinal complications and improve visual outcomes in patients with diabetes.

In conclusion, hyperglycemia exerts profound effects on retinal tissue, contributing to the pathogenesis of diabetic retinopathy through molecular, cellular, and structural mechanisms. Chronic exposure to elevated blood glucose levels induces oxidative stress, inflammation, vascular dysfunction, neurodegeneration, and functional impairment in the retina, leading to microvascular complications, neurovascular dysfunction, and vision loss in individuals with diabetes. Understanding the complex interplay between hyperglycemia and retinal pathology is essential for developing effective therapeutic strategies to preserve retinal function and prevent vision-threatening complications in diabetic retinopathy.

## Oxidative Stress and Antioxidant Mechanisms in Diabetic Retinopathy

Oxidative stress, characterized by an imbalance between the production of reactive oxygen species (ROS) and the antioxidant defense mechanisms, plays a central role in the pathogenesis of diabetic retinopathy (DR). Chronic hyperglycemia, the hallmark feature of diabetes mellitus, triggers oxidative stress in retinal tissues, leading to cellular damage, inflammation, and vascular dysfunction. Understanding the mechanisms underlying oxidative stress and antioxidant defense is crucial for elucidating the pathophysiology of DR and developing targeted therapeutic interventions to mitigate its progression.

### Oxidative Stress in Diabetic Retinopathy:

1. **ROS Production:** Hyperglycemia induces the production of ROS through various cellular pathways, including mitochondrial dysfunction, NADPH oxidase activation, and advanced glycation end product (AGE) formation. ROS, such as superoxide anion ($O2^{\cdot-}$), hydroxyl radical ($\cdot OH$), and hydrogen peroxide ($H2O2$), are highly reactive molecules that can damage cellular macromolecules, including lipids, proteins, and DNA.
2. **Lipid Peroxidation:** ROS attack and oxidize polyunsaturated fatty acids in cell membranes, leading to lipid peroxidation and the formation of reactive lipid species, such as malondialdehyde (MDA) and 4-hydroxynonenal (4-HNE). Lipid peroxidation products can

disrupt membrane integrity, alter membrane fluidity, and impair cellular function, contributing to retinal cell damage and dysfunction in DR.

3. **Protein Oxidation:** ROS react with amino acid residues in proteins, leading to protein oxidation, carbonylation, and nitrosylation. Protein oxidation alters protein structure and function, impairing enzymatic activity, receptor signaling, and cytoskeletal organization in retinal cells. Oxidatively modified proteins accumulate in retinal tissues and contribute to neurovascular dysfunction and inflammation in DR.

4. **DNA Damage:** ROS induce oxidative damage to DNA, leading to the formation of DNA adducts, strand breaks, and base modifications. DNA damage activates repair mechanisms, such as base excision repair and nucleotide excision repair, which can be overwhelmed under conditions of chronic oxidative stress. Accumulation of unrepaired DNA damage can lead to mutagenesis, cell cycle arrest, and apoptosis in retinal cells, exacerbating retinal degeneration in DR.

**Antioxidant Defense Mechanisms:**

1. **Enzymatic Antioxidants:**
   - **Superoxide Dismutase (SOD):** SOD catalyzes the dismutation of superoxide radicals ($O_2^{\cdot-}$) into molecular oxygen ($O_2$) and hydrogen peroxide ($H_2O_2$), reducing the levels of superoxide and preventing its conversion to more reactive ROS.
   - **Catalase (CAT):** Catalase converts hydrogen peroxide ($H_2O_2$) into water ($H_2O$) and molecular oxygen ($O_2$), neutralizing this potentially harmful ROS and protecting cells from oxidative damage.
   - **Glutathione Peroxidase (GPx):** GPx utilizes reduced glutathione (GSH) as a cofactor to

detoxify hydrogen peroxide (H2O2) and lipid hydroperoxides, reducing oxidative stress and maintaining cellular redox homeostasis.

2. **Non-enzymatic Antioxidants:**
   - **Glutathione (GSH):** GSH is a tripeptide antioxidant that serves as a cofactor for GPx and acts as a direct scavenger of ROS, neutralizing free radicals and protecting cellular components from oxidative damage.
   - **Vitamin C (Ascorbic Acid):** Vitamin C is a water-soluble antioxidant that scavenges ROS and regenerates other antioxidants, such as vitamin E, from their oxidized forms, thereby enhancing the overall antioxidant capacity of the cell.
   - **Vitamin E (α-Tocopherol):** Vitamin E is a lipid-soluble antioxidant that protects cell membranes from lipid peroxidation by scavenging lipid radicals and inhibiting the propagation of oxidative chain reactions.

**Dysregulation of Antioxidant Defense in Diabetic Retinopathy:**

1. **Reduced Antioxidant Enzyme Activity:** Chronic hyperglycemia and oxidative stress impair the activity of antioxidant enzymes, such as SOD, CAT, and GPx, in retinal tissues. Reduced enzyme activity compromises the ability of cells to neutralize ROS and detoxify oxidative intermediates, exacerbating oxidative damage and inflammation in DR.

2. **Depletion of Non-enzymatic Antioxidants:** Prolonged exposure to elevated ROS levels depletes non-enzymatic antioxidants, such as GSH, vitamin C, and vitamin E, in retinal tissues. Depletion of antioxidants impairs cellular defense mechanisms against oxidative stress, rendering retinal cells more susceptible to oxidative damage and

apoptosis in DR.

3. **Altered Redox Signaling Pathways:** Dysregulation of redox signaling pathways in response to oxidative stress contributes to retinal inflammation, neurodegeneration, and angiogenesis in DR. ROS serve as signaling molecules that modulate gene expression, protein function, and cellular responses to stress, influencing the progression of retinal pathology in diabetes.

**Therapeutic Implications:**

Targeting oxidative stress and antioxidant defense mechanisms represents a promising therapeutic approach for the management of diabetic retinopathy. Pharmacological agents that enhance antioxidant enzyme activity, replenish non-enzymatic antioxidants, and modulate redox signaling pathways may help mitigate oxidative damage and inflammation in retinal tissues. Additionally, lifestyle modifications, such as dietary antioxidants, regular exercise, and smoking cessation, may support endogenous antioxidant defense mechanisms and reduce the risk of retinal complications in diabetes.

In conclusion, oxidative stress plays a pivotal role in the pathogenesis of diabetic retinopathy, contributing to retinal damage, inflammation, and vascular dysfunction. Chronic hyperglycemia induces the production of reactive oxygen species (ROS) and impairs antioxidant defense mechanisms in retinal tissues, leading to cellular injury, neurovascular dysfunction, and vision loss in diabetes. Understanding the molecular mechanisms underlying oxidative stress and antioxidant regulation is essential for developing targeted therapeutic interventions to preserve retinal function and prevent vision-threatening complications in diabetic retinopathy.

## Inflammation and Immune Response in Diabetic Retinopathy

Inflammation and immune dysregulation play crucial roles in the pathogenesis of diabetic retinopathy (DR), a sight-threatening complication of diabetes mellitus. Chronic hyperglycemia triggers a cascade of inflammatory responses within the retina, leading to endothelial dysfunction, leukocyte infiltration, and retinal tissue damage. Understanding the mechanisms underlying inflammation and immune activation in DR is essential for elucidating its pathophysiology and developing targeted therapeutic strategies to prevent or mitigate its progression.

## Inflammatory Mediators in Diabetic Retinopathy:

1. **Pro-inflammatory Cytokines:** Elevated levels of pro-inflammatory cytokines, such as tumor necrosis factor-alpha (TNF-α), interleukin-1 beta (IL-1β), and interleukin-6 (IL-6), are observed in the vitreous and aqueous humor of patients with DR. These cytokines contribute to endothelial activation, leukocyte recruitment, and vascular permeability, promoting the development of retinal microvascular abnormalities and macular edema in DR.

2. **Chemokines and Adhesion Molecules:** Chemokines, such as monocyte chemoattractant protein-1 (MCP-1) and interleukin-8 (IL-8), facilitate the recruitment of leukocytes, including monocytes and neutrophils, to the retina in response to hyperglycemia-induced inflammation. Adhesion molecules, such as intercellular adhesion molecule-1 (ICAM-1) and vascular cell adhesion molecule-1 (VCAM-1), mediate the adhesion and transendothelial migration of leukocytes across the blood-

retinal barrier, exacerbating retinal inflammation and tissue damage in DR.

3. **Oxidative Stress and Inflammatory Signaling:** Oxidative stress, induced by chronic hyperglycemia, amplifies inflammatory signaling pathways in the retina, leading to the activation of nuclear factor-kappa B (NF-κB) and mitogen-activated protein kinase (MAPK) pathways. These pathways regulate the expression of pro-inflammatory genes, such as cyclooxygenase-2 (COX-2) and inducible nitric oxide synthase (iNOS), and promote the production of ROS and reactive nitrogen species (RNS), perpetuating retinal inflammation and oxidative damage in DR.

**Cellular Players in Retinal Inflammation:**

1. **Microglia and Macrophages:** Resident microglial cells and infiltrating macrophages are key players in retinal inflammation and immune response in DR. Activated microglia/macrophages release pro-inflammatory cytokines, phagocytose damaged cells and debris, and contribute to vascular dysfunction and neurodegeneration in the diabetic retina. Microglial/ macrophage activation is observed in early stages of DR and correlates with disease severity and progression.

2. **Endothelial Cells:** Retinal endothelial cells respond to inflammatory stimuli by upregulating adhesion molecules, such as ICAM-1 and VCAM-1, and secreting chemokines that promote leukocyte recruitment and vascular permeability. Endothelial dysfunction, characterized by impaired nitric oxide bioavailability and increased production of vasoconstrictors, contributes to capillary dropout, ischemia, and neovascularization in advanced stages of DR.

3. **Müller Cells and Astrocytes:** Müller cells and astrocytes, glial cells that provide structural and metabolic support to retinal neurons and blood vessels, participate in retinal

inflammation and immune response in DR. Activated Müller cells and astrocytes upregulate inflammatory mediators, such as cytokines and chemokines, and contribute to the breakdown of the blood-retinal barrier, exacerbating retinal edema and neurovascular dysfunction in DR.

**Immune-Mediated Pathways in Diabetic Retinopathy:**

1. **Innate Immune Response:** The innate immune system plays a critical role in the initiation and propagation of retinal inflammation in DR. Toll-like receptors (TLRs), pattern recognition receptors expressed on retinal cells, recognize pathogen-associated molecular patterns (PAMPs) and damage-associated molecular patterns (DAMPs) released in response to hyperglycemia-induced stress and injury. Activation of TLR signaling pathways triggers the production of pro-inflammatory cytokines and chemokines, amplifying retinal inflammation and tissue damage in DR.

2. **Adaptive Immune Response:** Growing evidence suggests the involvement of adaptive immune mechanisms, including T lymphocytes and B lymphocytes, in the pathogenesis of DR. Infiltration of activated T cells into the retina promotes local inflammation and tissue damage, while dysregulation of T cell subsets, such as Th1, Th17, and Treg cells, contributes to the imbalance between pro-inflammatory and anti-inflammatory responses in DR. B lymphocytes produce antibodies and cytokines that modulate immune responses and promote tissue damage in the diabetic retina.

**Therapeutic Implications:**

Targeting inflammation and immune dysregulation represents a promising therapeutic approach for the management of diabetic retinopathy. Pharmacological agents that inhibit pro-inflammatory cytokines, block leukocyte adhesion and migration, and modulate immune cell activation may help mitigate retinal inflammation and vascular dysfunction in DR. Additionally, lifestyle modifications, such as diet, exercise, and smoking cessation, may modulate systemic inflammation and reduce the risk of retinal complications in diabetes.

In conclusion, inflammation and immune dysregulation play critical roles in the pathogenesis of diabetic retinopathy, contributing to retinal vascular dysfunction, neurodegeneration, and vision loss in diabetes. Chronic hyperglycemia induces the production of inflammatory mediators, such as cytokines, chemokines, and adhesion molecules, and activates innate and adaptive immune responses in the retina, perpetuating retinal inflammation and tissue damage in DR. Understanding the molecular mechanisms underlying retinal inflammation and immune activation is essential for developing targeted therapeutic interventions to prevent or mitigate the progression of diabetic retinopathy and preserve vision in individuals with diabetes.

# CHAPTER 4: CLINICAL MANIFESTATIONS OF DIABETIC RETINOPATHY

## Non-Proliferative Diabetic Retinopathy (NPDR)

Non-proliferative diabetic retinopathy (NPDR) is an early stage of diabetic retinopathy (DR) characterized by microvascular abnormalities, retinal hemorrhages, and lipid exudates in the absence of neovascularization. NPDR represents the initial phase of retinal pathology in diabetes mellitus and serves as a precursor to more severe stages of DR, including proliferative diabetic retinopathy (PDR) and diabetic macular edema (DME). Understanding the clinical features, pathophysiology, and management of NPDR is essential for early detection, risk stratification, and timely intervention to prevent vision-threatening complications in individuals with diabetes.

## Clinical Features of Non-Proliferative Diabetic Retinopathy:

1. **Microaneurysms:** Microaneurysms are small outpouchings of retinal capillaries that result from focal

weakening of the vessel wall. They appear as red dots on fundus examination and are the earliest clinically visible sign of NPDR. Microaneurysms are prone to leakage, leading to retinal hemorrhages and lipid exudates.

2. **Retinal Hemorrhages:** Retinal hemorrhages manifest as dot or blot hemorrhages on fundus examination and result from the rupture of retinal capillaries. They are often distributed along the retinal vessels and may vary in size and severity. Retinal hemorrhages are indicative of microvascular damage and increased vascular permeability in NPDR.

3. **Hard Exudates:** Hard exudates are yellow-white deposits of lipids and proteins that accumulate in the outer plexiform layer of the retina. They typically occur adjacent to areas of capillary leakage and represent lipid leakage from damaged retinal vessels. Hard exudates are a hallmark feature of diabetic macular edema (DME) and are associated with vision loss and macular thickening.

4. **Cotton Wool Spots:** Cotton wool spots, also known as soft exudates, are focal areas of retinal ischemia and nerve fiber layer infarction. They appear as fluffy white lesions on fundus examination and result from microvascular occlusion and disruption of axoplasmic transport. Cotton wool spots are indicative of retinal hypoxia and neurovascular dysfunction in NPDR.

5. **Intraretinal Microvascular Abnormalities (IRMAs):** IRMAs are tortuous and dilated retinal vessels that develop as compensatory mechanisms in response to retinal ischemia and capillary non-perfusion. They represent areas of retinal neovascularization and are more commonly observed in advanced stages of NPDR.

**Pathophysiology of Non-Proliferative Diabetic Retinopathy:**

1. **Microvascular Damage:** Chronic hyperglycemia and metabolic dysregulation lead to endothelial dysfunction

and microvascular damage in the retina. Increased oxidative stress, inflammation, and formation of advanced glycation end products (AGEs) contribute to the breakdown of the blood-retinal barrier (BRB) and disruption of retinal vascular homeostasis.

2. **Capillary Leakage:** Impaired endothelial function and increased vascular permeability result in the leakage of plasma proteins, lipids, and inflammatory mediators into the retinal tissue. Capillary leakage leads to the formation of microaneurysms, retinal hemorrhages, and lipid exudates characteristic of NPDR. Leakage of fluid and lipids into the macula can cause macular edema and vision loss.

3. **Ischemia and Hypoxia:** Microvascular occlusion and capillary dropout lead to retinal ischemia and hypoxia in areas of non-perfusion. Hypoxic retinal tissue releases angiogenic factors, such as vascular endothelial growth factor (VEGF), that promote neovascularization and fibrovascular proliferation in advanced stages of DR.

4. **Neurovascular Dysfunction:** Retinal neurovascular dysfunction, characterized by impaired neurovascular coupling and neuronal apoptosis, contributes to the pathogenesis of NPDR. Hypoxia-induced retinal ganglion cell (RGC) death and dysfunction of Müller cells and astrocytes impair retinal function and exacerbate neurovascular damage in diabetes.

## Management of Non-Proliferative Diabetic Retinopathy:

1. **Optimized Glycemic Control:** Tight glycemic control is essential for preventing and managing NPDR in individuals with diabetes. Intensive glucose-lowering therapy reduces the risk of microvascular complications and slows the progression of retinal pathology in diabetes. Patients should undergo regular monitoring of blood glucose levels and hemoglobin A1c (HbA1c) to optimize

glycemic control and minimize the risk of DR progression.

2. **Blood Pressure Management:** Systemic hypertension is a major risk factor for NPDR and other microvascular complications in diabetes. Blood pressure control, through lifestyle modifications and antihypertensive medications, helps preserve retinal vascular integrity and reduce the risk of retinal hemorrhages, exudates, and neovascularization in NPDR.

3. **Lifestyle Modifications:** Lifestyle interventions, including smoking cessation, dietary modifications, regular exercise, and weight management, are important for preventing and managing NPDR in individuals with diabetes. Smoking cessation reduces oxidative stress and improves retinal vascular function, while a healthy diet and regular exercise promote metabolic health and reduce the risk of microvascular complications.

4. **Ocular Screening and Monitoring:** Regular ocular screening and monitoring are essential for early detection and management of NPDR in individuals with diabetes. Dilated fundus examination, optical coherence tomography (OCT), and fundus photography are used to assess retinal morphology, detect microvascular abnormalities, and monitor disease progression over time.

5. **Pharmacological Interventions:** Pharmacological interventions, including intravitreal anti-VEGF therapy, intravitreal corticosteroid injections, and laser photocoagulation, may be indicated for the management of NPDR-associated complications, such as diabetic macular edema (DME) and vision-threatening retinal neovascularization. Anti-VEGF agents reduce vascular leakage and inhibit neovascularization, while corticosteroids reduce inflammation and edema in the macula.

In summary, non-proliferative diabetic retinopathy (NPDR) is an early stage of diabetic retinopathy characterized by microvascular abnormalities, retinal hemorrhages, and lipid exudates. NPDR represents the initial phase of retinal pathology in diabetes and serves as a precursor to more severe stages of DR. Chronic hyperglycemia and metabolic dysregulation lead to endothelial dysfunction, capillary leakage, and retinal ischemia, contributing to the pathogenesis of NPDR. Early detection, risk stratification, and timely intervention are essential for preventing vision-threatening complications in individuals with NPDR. Management strategies for NPDR include optimized glycemic control, blood pressure management, lifestyle modifications, ocular screening, and pharmacological interventions to preserve retinal function and minimize disease progression in diabetes.

## Proliferative Diabetic Retinopathy (PDR)

Proliferative diabetic retinopathy (PDR) represents an advanced stage of diabetic retinopathy (DR) characterized by the growth of abnormal retinal blood vessels, termed neovascularization, on the surface of the retina and optic disc. PDR is a sight-threatening complication of diabetes mellitus and is associated with an increased risk of vitreous hemorrhage, tractional retinal detachment, and neovascular glaucoma. Understanding the clinical features, pathophysiology, and management of PDR is crucial for early detection, risk stratification, and timely intervention to prevent irreversible vision loss in individuals with diabetes.

### Clinical Features of Proliferative Diabetic Retinopathy:

1. **Neovascularization:** Neovascularization is the hallmark feature of PDR and manifests as fine, delicate vessels on the surface of the retina, optic disc, and posterior hyaloid membrane. Neovascularization arises from areas of retinal

ischemia and hypoxia and extends into the vitreous cavity, where it is prone to hemorrhage and fibrovascular proliferation.

2. **Vitreous Hemorrhage:** Neovascularization in PDR can lead to the formation of fragile, leaky blood vessels that are susceptible to rupture and bleeding. Vitreous hemorrhage occurs when neovascular vessels bleed into the vitreous cavity, causing sudden vision loss or floaters. Vitreous hemorrhage may resolve spontaneously or require surgical intervention, depending on its severity and duration.

3. **Tractional Retinal Detachment:** PDR is often associated with the development of fibrovascular membranes on the retinal surface, which contract and exert tractional forces on the retina. Tractional retinal detachment occurs when fibrovascular membranes pull on the retina, leading to its separation from the underlying retinal pigment epithelium (RPE) and choroid. Tractional retinal detachment can cause visual distortion, peripheral visual field loss, and permanent vision loss if left untreated.

4. **Neovascular Glaucoma:** Neovascularization of the anterior segment of the eye, particularly the iris and angle structures, can lead to neovascular glaucoma in individuals with PDR. Neovascular glaucoma is characterized by elevated intraocular pressure (IOP) due to the obstruction of aqueous outflow by neovascular membranes. Neovascular glaucoma is difficult to manage and often requires aggressive treatment to control IOP and prevent optic nerve damage.

## Pathophysiology of Proliferative Diabetic Retinopathy:

1. **Ischemia-Driven Angiogenesis:** Chronic hyperglycemia and metabolic dysregulation lead to retinal ischemia and hypoxia, triggering the release of angiogenic factors, such as vascular endothelial growth factor (VEGF) and fibroblast growth factor (FGF), from ischemic retinal

cells. Angiogenic factors promote the proliferation and migration of endothelial cells, leading to the formation of abnormal retinal blood vessels characteristic of PDR.

2. **Fibrovascular Proliferation:** Neovascularization in PDR is accompanied by fibrovascular proliferation, characterized by the infiltration of fibroblasts, myofibroblasts, and extracellular matrix proteins into the retinal tissue. Fibrovascular membranes contract and exert tractional forces on the retina, leading to the formation of preretinal fibrous bands and tractional retinal detachment in advanced stages of PDR.

3. **Inflammatory and Immune Responses:** Inflammatory mediators and immune cells contribute to the pathogenesis of PDR by promoting angiogenesis, fibrovascular proliferation, and tissue remodeling in the diabetic retina. Inflammatory cytokines, such as tumor necrosis factor-alpha (TNF-α) and interleukin-6 (IL-6), stimulate endothelial cell activation and VEGF production, exacerbating neovascularization and vascular leakage in PDR.

4. **Neurovascular Crosstalk:** Retinal neurovascular dysfunction, characterized by impaired neurovascular coupling and neuronal apoptosis, influences the progression of PDR. Hypoxia-induced retinal ganglion cell (RGC) death and dysfunction of Müller cells and astrocytes exacerbate retinal ischemia and neovascularization in diabetes. Neurovascular crosstalk between retinal neurons, glial cells, and vascular endothelium contributes to the pathogenesis of PDR and influences its clinical manifestations.

## Management of Proliferative Diabetic Retinopathy:

1. **Panretinal Photocoagulation (PRP):** Panretinal photocoagulation is the standard treatment for PDR and aims to reduce retinal ischemia and VEGF production

by ablating ischemic retinal tissue. PRP involves the application of laser burns to the peripheral retina, targeting areas of non-perfusion and neovascularization. PRP reduces the risk of vision-threatening complications, such as vitreous hemorrhage and tractional retinal detachment, and preserves central vision in individuals with PDR.

2. **Intravitreal Anti-VEGF Therapy:** Intravitreal injection of anti-VEGF agents, such as ranibizumab, bevacizumab, and aflibercept, is an effective treatment option for PDR-associated complications, such as diabetic macular edema (DME) and neovascular glaucoma. Anti-VEGF therapy inhibits VEGF-mediated angiogenesis and vascular leakage, reducing the risk of vision loss and improving visual outcomes in individuals with PDR.

3. **Vitrectomy Surgery:** Vitrectomy surgery is indicated for the management of severe complications of PDR, such as non-clearing vitreous hemorrhage, tractional retinal detachment, and macular traction. Vitrectomy involves the removal of vitreous hemorrhage, fibrovascular membranes, and tractional forces from the retinal surface, restoring retinal anatomy and preserving visual function in advanced stages of PDR.

4. **Adjunctive Therapies:** Adjunctive therapies, including corticosteroid implants, intravitreal anti-inflammatory agents, and anti-fibrotic agents, may be used in combination with laser photocoagulation or anti-VEGF therapy to enhance treatment outcomes and reduce the risk of PDR progression. Corticosteroids exert anti-inflammatory and anti-angiogenic effects, while anti-fibrotic agents inhibit fibrovascular proliferation and contraction in the diabetic retina.

5. **Ocular Screening and Monitoring:** Regular ocular screening and monitoring are essential for early detection and management of PDR in individuals with

diabetes. Dilated fundus examination, optical coherence tomography (OCT), and fluorescein angiography are used to assess retinal morphology, detect neovascularization, and monitor disease progression over time.

In conclusion, proliferative diabetic retinopathy (PDR) is an advanced stage of diabetic retinopathy characterized by the growth of abnormal retinal blood vessels and fibrovascular proliferation on the retinal surface. PDR is associated with an increased risk of vitreous hemorrhage, tractional retinal detachment, and neovascular glaucoma, leading to irreversible vision loss if left untreated. Chronic hyperglycemia, retinal ischemia, and inflammatory responses contribute to the pathogenesis of PDR, driving neovascularization and fibrovascular proliferation in the diabetic retina. Early detection, risk stratification, and timely intervention are essential for preserving visual function and preventing vision-threatening complications in individuals with PDR. Management strategies for PDR include panretinal photocoagulation, intravitreal anti-VEGF therapy, vitrectomy surgery, and adjunctive therapies to reduce retinal ischemia, inhibit angiogenesis, and restore retinal anatomy in advanced stages of the disease. Regular ocular screening and monitoring are essential for optimizing treatment outcomes and preserving vision in individuals with PDR.

## Diabetic Macular Edema (DME)

Diabetic macular edema (DME) is a common complication of diabetic retinopathy (DR) characterized by the accumulation of fluid in the macula, the central portion of the retina responsible for sharp, detailed vision. DME is a major cause of vision loss in individuals with diabetes mellitus and can significantly impair central visual acuity and quality of life. Understanding the clinical features, pathophysiology, and management of DME is essential for early detection, risk stratification, and timely intervention to preserve visual function and prevent irreversible vision loss in individuals with diabetes.

**Clinical Features of Diabetic Macular Edema:**

1. **Visual Disturbances:** DME can cause visual disturbances, such as blurriness, distortion, and central vision loss, that affect activities such as reading, driving, and recognizing faces. Visual symptoms may vary in severity and can significantly impact the quality of life of affected individuals.

2. **Macular Thickening:** DME is characterized by increased retinal thickness in the macula due to the accumulation of fluid in the retinal layers. Optical coherence tomography (OCT) imaging reveals cystoid spaces, intraretinal fluid, and subretinal fluid in the macular region, indicative of macular edema.

3. **Hard Exudates:** Lipid exudates, or hard exudates, may accumulate in the macula as a result of fluid leakage from damaged retinal vessels. Hard exudates appear as yellow-white deposits on fundus examination and are often distributed around areas of capillary leakage in DME.

4. **Reduced Visual Acuity:** DME can lead to a decrease in central visual acuity, affecting tasks that require detailed vision and visual acuity, such as reading fine print or recognizing faces. Visual acuity may fluctuate depending on the severity and duration of DME and the presence of comorbid ocular conditions.

**Pathophysiology of Diabetic Macular Edema:**

1. **Blood-Retinal Barrier Dysfunction:** Chronic hyperglycemia and metabolic dysregulation lead to endothelial dysfunction and breakdown of the blood-

retinal barrier (BRB) in the macula. Increased vascular permeability and leakage of plasma proteins, including albumin and lipoproteins, into the retinal tissue contribute to the formation of macular edema in DME.

2. **Inflammatory Mediators:** Inflammatory cytokines, such as tumor necrosis factor-alpha (TNF-α), interleukin-1 beta (IL-1β), and interleukin-6 (IL-6), are upregulated in the diabetic retina and contribute to the pathogenesis of DME. Inflammatory mediators promote endothelial activation, leukocyte recruitment, and vascular permeability, exacerbating macular edema and retinal tissue damage in DR.

3. **Vascular Endothelial Growth Factor (VEGF):** Vascular endothelial growth factor (VEGF) plays a central role in the pathogenesis of DME by promoting vascular permeability, angiogenesis, and inflammation in the diabetic retina. Elevated levels of VEGF are observed in the vitreous and aqueous humor of patients with DME and correlate with disease severity and visual impairment.

4. **Oxidative Stress:** Oxidative stress, characterized by an imbalance between the production of reactive oxygen species (ROS) and antioxidant defense mechanisms, contributes to the pathogenesis of DME. ROS induce endothelial dysfunction, inflammation, and vascular permeability in the diabetic retina, exacerbating macular edema and retinal tissue damage.

**Management of Diabetic Macular Edema:**

1. **Intravitreal Anti-VEGF Therapy:** Intravitreal injection of anti-VEGF agents, such as ranibizumab, bevacizumab, and aflibercept, is the first-line treatment for DME and aims to reduce macular edema and improve visual acuity. Anti-VEGF therapy inhibits VEGF-mediated angiogenesis and vascular leakage, promoting the resolution of macular edema and restoring retinal architecture.

2. **Intravitreal Corticosteroid Therapy:** Intravitreal injection of corticosteroids, such as triamcinolone acetonide and dexamethasone, is an alternative treatment option for DME, particularly in cases resistant to anti-VEGF therapy. Corticosteroids exert anti-inflammatory and anti-angiogenic effects, reducing macular edema and improving visual acuity in individuals with DME.

3. **Focal/Grid Laser Photocoagulation:** Focal/grid laser photocoagulation is a longstanding treatment modality for DME that aims to reduce macular edema and stabilize visual acuity. Laser photocoagulation targets microaneurysms, areas of capillary leakage, and ischemic retinal tissue to promote retinal remodeling and reduce vascular permeability in the macula.

4. **Vitrectomy Surgery:** Vitrectomy surgery may be indicated for the management of severe or refractory DME associated with tractional retinal detachment, epiretinal membrane formation, or vitreomacular traction. Vitrectomy involves the removal of vitreous gel, fibrovascular membranes, and tractional forces from the retinal surface, restoring retinal anatomy and improving visual function in advanced cases of DME.

5. **Ocular Screening and Monitoring:** Regular ocular screening and monitoring are essential for early detection and management of DME in individuals with diabetes. Dilated fundus examination, optical coherence tomography (OCT), and fluorescein angiography are used to assess macular morphology, detect macular edema, and monitor treatment response over time.

In summary, diabetic macular edema (DME) is a common complication of diabetic retinopathy characterized by the accumulation of fluid in the macula, leading to visual disturbances and central vision loss. Chronic hyperglycemia, vascular endothelial dysfunction, and inflammatory mediators contribute to the pathogenesis of DME by promoting macular edema and retinal tissue damage. Early detection, risk stratification, and timely intervention are essential for preserving visual function and preventing irreversible vision loss in individuals with DME. Management strategies for DME include intravitreal anti-VEGF therapy, intravitreal corticosteroid therapy, laser photocoagulation, vitrectomy surgery, and regular ocular screening to optimize treatment outcomes and preserve vision in diabetes.

## Other Complications: Neovascular Glaucoma and Vitreous Hemorrhage

In addition to diabetic macular edema (DME) and proliferative diabetic retinopathy (PDR), individuals with diabetes mellitus are at risk of developing other sight-threatening complications, including neovascular glaucoma (NVG) and vitreous hemorrhage. These complications can lead to irreversible vision loss if left untreated and require prompt diagnosis and intervention to preserve visual function and prevent further ocular damage.

### Neovascular Glaucoma (NVG):

Neovascular glaucoma is a secondary form of glaucoma characterized by elevated intraocular pressure (IOP) due to the growth of abnormal blood vessels on the iris and angle structures of the eye. NVG typically arises as a complication of advanced proliferative diabetic retinopathy (PDR) or ischemic retinal conditions and is associated with poor visual outcomes and high rates of blindness if left untreated.

### Clinical Features of Neovascular Glaucoma:

1. **Elevated Intraocular Pressure (IOP):** Elevated IOP is the

hallmark feature of neovascular glaucoma and results from the obstruction of aqueous outflow by abnormal blood vessels on the iris and angle structures. Increased IOP can cause optic nerve damage and visual field loss if not controlled promptly.

2. **Neovascularization of the Iris (NVI):** Neovascularization of the iris, characterized by the growth of fine, delicate blood vessels on the iris surface, is a key diagnostic feature of NVG. NVI is often associated with areas of retinal ischemia and neovascularization in proliferative diabetic retinopathy (PDR) and indicates severe ocular ischemia and vascular dysfunction.

3. **Conjunctival Injection:** Conjunctival injection, or redness of the conjunctiva, may be observed in individuals with neovascular glaucoma due to the presence of abnormal blood vessels on the iris and angle structures. Conjunctival injection is often associated with ocular pain, discomfort, and photophobia in NVG.

4. **Corneal Edema:** Corneal edema, characterized by clouding and swelling of the cornea, may occur secondary to elevated intraocular pressure (IOP) and compromised corneal endothelial function in neovascular glaucoma. Corneal edema can lead to visual impairment and discomfort in affected individuals.

**Management of Neovascular Glaucoma:**

1. **Intraocular Pressure Control:** The primary goal of neovascular glaucoma management is to reduce intraocular pressure (IOP) and prevent optic nerve damage and visual field loss. Topical and systemic ocular hypotensive medications, such as beta-blockers, prostaglandin analogs, and carbonic anhydrase inhibitors, may be used to lower IOP and control glaucoma progression.

2. **Anti-VEGF Therapy:** Intravitreal injection of anti-vascular

endothelial growth factor (anti-VEGF) agents, such as ranibizumab and bevacizumab, may be indicated for the management of neovascular glaucoma associated with proliferative diabetic retinopathy (PDR). Anti-VEGF therapy inhibits angiogenesis and vascular leakage, reducing neovascularization and ocular inflammation in NVG.

3. **Panretinal Photocoagulation (PRP):** Panretinal photocoagulation is the standard treatment for proliferative diabetic retinopathy (PDR) and may be indicated for the management of neovascular glaucoma associated with retinal ischemia. PRP reduces retinal ischemia and VEGF production, leading to regression of abnormal blood vessels and stabilization of intraocular pressure (IOP) in NVG.

4. **Cyclophotocoagulation:** Transscleral cyclophotocoagulation, or laser cycloablation, may be considered as a treatment option for refractory neovascular glaucoma that is unresponsive to medical therapy and conventional laser treatments. Cyclophotocoagulation targets the ciliary body, reducing aqueous humor production and lowering intraocular pressure (IOP) in NVG.

## Vitreous Hemorrhage:

Vitreous hemorrhage is a common complication of diabetic retinopathy characterized by the leakage of blood into the vitreous cavity from abnormal retinal blood vessels. Vitreous hemorrhage can cause sudden vision loss or floaters and may be associated with proliferative diabetic retinopathy (PDR) or retinal tears and detachments.

## Clinical Features of Vitreous Hemorrhage:

1. **Sudden Vision Loss:** Vitreous hemorrhage can cause sudden and profound vision loss due to the obstruction

of light transmission through the vitreous cavity. Visual acuity may range from mildly decreased to hand motion or light perception only, depending on the extent and location of hemorrhage.

2. **Floaters and Spots:** Floaters, or dark spots and specks in the visual field, may be observed by individuals with vitreous hemorrhage due to the presence of blood cells suspended in the vitreous gel. Floaters may interfere with visual function and reduce visual acuity in affected individuals.

3. **Retinal Detachment:** Vitreous hemorrhage may be associated with retinal tears or detachments, particularly in cases of proliferative diabetic retinopathy (PDR) or tractional retinal detachment. Retinal detachment can cause peripheral visual field loss, photopsia, and visual distortion, indicating a need for urgent surgical intervention.

**Management of Vitreous Hemorrhage:**

1. **Observation and Monitoring:** Mild to moderate vitreous hemorrhage may resolve spontaneously over time without intervention, particularly in cases of non-proliferative diabetic retinopathy (NPDR) or non-tractional hemorrhage. Close observation and monitoring of visual symptoms and retinal morphology are essential for determining the need for further intervention.

2. **Vitrectomy Surgery:** Vitrectomy surgery is indicated for the management of severe or persistent vitreous hemorrhage associated with proliferative diabetic retinopathy (PDR), tractional retinal detachment, or non-clearing hemorrhage. Vitrectomy involves the removal of vitreous gel and blood from the vitreous cavity, allowing visualization and treatment of retinal pathology.

3. **Panretinal Photocoagulation (PRP):** Panretinal photocoagulation may be performed in conjunction

with vitrectomy surgery for the management of vitreous hemorrhage associated with proliferative diabetic retinopathy (PDR). PRP reduces retinal ischemia and VEGF production, promoting regression of abnormal blood vessels and stabilization of retinal vasculature.

4. **Anti-VEGF Therapy:** Intravitreal injection of anti-vascular endothelial growth factor (anti-VEGF) agents may be considered as an adjunctive treatment for vitreous hemorrhage associated with proliferative diabetic retinopathy (PDR). Anti-VEGF therapy inhibits angiogenesis and vascular leakage, reducing the risk of recurrent hemorrhage and promoting retinal healing and stabilization.

In summary, neovascular glaucoma (NVG) and vitreous hemorrhage are sight-threatening complications of diabetic retinopathy (DR) that require prompt diagnosis and intervention to preserve visual function and prevent irreversible vision loss in individuals with diabetes. Neovascular glaucoma is characterized by elevated intraocular pressure (IOP) and neovascularization of the iris and angle structures, while vitreous hemorrhage is characterized by the leakage of blood into the vitreous cavity from abnormal retinal blood vessels. Management strategies for NVG and vitreous hemorrhage include intraocular pressure control, anti-VEGF therapy, panretinal photocoagulation, vitrectomy surgery, and close observation and monitoring of visual symptoms and retinal morphology. Early detection, risk stratification, and timely intervention are essential for optimizing treatment outcomes and preserving visual function in individuals with diabetes mellitus.

# CHAPTER 5: DIAGNOSTIC TECHNIQUES

## Fundoscopic Examination

Fundoscopic examination, also known as ophthalmoscopy or fundoscopy, is a crucial diagnostic tool used by healthcare professionals to assess the health and integrity of the retina, optic disc, and posterior segment of the eye. In the context of diabetic retinopathy (DR), fundoscopic examination plays a pivotal role in the early detection, diagnosis, and monitoring of retinal pathology associated with diabetes mellitus. This section provides an overview of fundoscopic examination techniques, findings, and their significance in the evaluation of diabetic retinopathy.

## Techniques of Fundoscopic Examination:

1. **Direct Ophthalmoscopy:** Direct ophthalmoscopy involves the use of a handheld ophthalmoscope to visualize the posterior segment of the eye, including the retina, optic disc, and macula. The examiner holds the ophthalmoscope close to the patient's eye and shines a beam of light into

the pupil while observing the fundus through the device's viewing aperture.

2. **Indirect Ophthalmoscopy:** Indirect ophthalmoscopy utilizes a condensing lens and a light source to provide a wider field of view of the fundus compared to direct ophthalmoscopy. The examiner holds the condensing lens in front of the patient's eye and views the inverted and magnified image of the fundus through the lens, allowing for a comprehensive examination of the retina and peripheral retina.

3. **Biomicroscopic Examination:** Biomicroscopic examination, also known as slit-lamp biomicroscopy, combines a slit lamp microscope with a biomicroscope to visualize the anterior and posterior segments of the eye in detail. The examiner adjusts the slit lamp beam to illuminate specific areas of the retina and uses various magnification lenses to examine retinal structures and pathology.

## Findings on Fundoscopic Examination in Diabetic Retinopathy:

1. **Microaneurysms:** Microaneurysms are small outpouchings of retinal capillaries that appear as round, red dots on fundoscopic examination. They are an early sign of diabetic retinopathy and indicate localized vascular abnormalities and microvascular damage in the retina.

2. **Hemorrhages:** Retinal hemorrhages manifest as dot or blot hemorrhages on fundoscopic examination and result from the rupture of retinal capillaries. Hemorrhages may be scattered throughout the retina and vary in size and severity depending on the extent of retinal ischemia and vascular pathology.

3. **Hard Exudates:** Hard exudates are yellow-white deposits of lipids and proteins that accumulate in the outer plexiform layer of the retina. They appear as well-defined, yellowish lesions on fundoscopic examination and are

often distributed around areas of capillary leakage and microaneurysms in diabetic retinopathy.

4. **Cotton Wool Spots:** Cotton wool spots, also known as soft exudates, are focal areas of retinal ischemia and nerve fiber layer infarction. They appear as fluffy white lesions on fundoscopic examination and result from microvascular occlusion and disruption of axoplasmic transport in the diabetic retina.

5. **Neovascularization:** Neovascularization is the growth of abnormal retinal blood vessels on the surface of the retina, optic disc, and posterior hyaloid membrane. It appears as fine, delicate vessels on fundoscopic examination and is a hallmark feature of proliferative diabetic retinopathy (PDR) and advanced stages of diabetic retinopathy.

6. **Macular Edema:** Macular edema is characterized by the accumulation of fluid in the macula, the central portion of the retina responsible for sharp, detailed vision. It may manifest as retinal thickening, cystoid spaces, and subretinal fluid on fundoscopic examination, indicating impaired retinal vascular integrity and increased vascular permeability.

**Significance of Fundoscopic Examination in Diabetic Retinopathy:**

1. **Early Detection and Diagnosis:** Fundoscopic examination enables the early detection and diagnosis of diabetic retinopathy by identifying characteristic retinal lesions and vascular abnormalities associated with diabetes mellitus. Early intervention and management are essential for preventing vision-threatening complications and preserving visual function in individuals with diabetic retinopathy.

2. **Assessment of Disease Severity:** Fundoscopic examination allows for the assessment of disease

severity and progression in diabetic retinopathy by evaluating the presence and extent of retinal pathology, including microaneurysms, hemorrhages, exudates, and neovascularization. The severity of retinal findings on fundoscopy correlates with the risk of vision loss and the need for treatment in diabetic retinopathy.

3. **Monitoring of Treatment Response:** Fundoscopic examination is essential for monitoring treatment response and disease progression in diabetic retinopathy following intervention, such as laser photocoagulation, intravitreal injections, or vitrectomy surgery. Serial fundoscopic evaluations enable healthcare professionals to assess the efficacy of treatment and adjust management strategies accordingly to optimize visual outcomes.

4. **Patient Education and Counseling:** Fundoscopic examination provides visual evidence of retinal pathology and vascular changes associated with diabetes mellitus, facilitating patient education and counseling about the importance of glycemic control, blood pressure management, and regular ocular screening in the prevention and management of diabetic retinopathy. Visual representation of retinal findings on fundoscopy enhances patient understanding and adherence to treatment recommendations.

In summary, fundoscopic examination is a fundamental component of the clinical evaluation and management of diabetic retinopathy, enabling the early detection, diagnosis, and monitoring of retinal pathology associated with diabetes mellitus. Direct and indirect ophthalmoscopy, as well as biomicroscopic examination, allow healthcare professionals to visualize characteristic retinal lesions, hemorrhages, exudates, and neovascularization in diabetic retinopathy and assess disease severity and treatment response. Fundoscopic examination plays a crucial role in guiding therapeutic decisions, monitoring disease progression, and optimizing visual outcomes in individuals with diabetes mellitus. Regular ocular screening and comprehensive fundoscopic evaluation are essential for the timely identification and management of diabetic retinopathy to prevent vision loss and preserve visual function in affected individuals.

## Optical Coherence Tomography (OCT)

Optical coherence tomography (OCT) is a non-invasive imaging technique that provides high-resolution, cross-sectional images of ocular structures, including the retina, retinal layers, and optic nerve head. In the context of diabetic retinopathy (DR), OCT plays a crucial role in the diagnosis, monitoring, and management of macular edema, retinal thickness changes, and structural abnormalities associated with diabetes mellitus. This section provides an overview of OCT principles, applications, and significance in the evaluation of diabetic retinopathy.

### Principles of Optical Coherence Tomography (OCT):

1. **Interferometry:** OCT utilizes low-coherence interferometry to generate cross-sectional images of ocular structures by measuring the interference patterns of backscattered light from tissue. A broadband light source is used to emit near-infrared light, which is split into a reference beam and a sample beam. The reference beam is directed to a reference mirror, while the sample beam is directed to the eye and focused on the retina. The interference between the reflected sample beam and the reference beam is detected and analyzed to reconstruct high-resolution, depth-resolved images of the retina.

2. **Depth Resolution:** OCT achieves high axial resolution by measuring the time delay or optical path length difference between the reference and sample beams, allowing for

precise localization of retinal structures and identification of subtle changes in tissue morphology. The depth resolution of OCT is determined by the coherence length of the light source and can range from a few micrometers to tens of micrometers, depending on the wavelength of light used.

3. **Cross-sectional Imaging:** OCT generates cross-sectional images, or B-scans, of the retina by scanning the sample beam across the retinal surface in a raster pattern. Each A-scan represents the intensity of backscattered light as a function of depth, allowing for visualization of retinal layers, thickness measurements, and identification of structural abnormalities.

## Applications of Optical Coherence Tomography (OCT) in Diabetic Retinopathy:

1. **Macular Edema Detection:** OCT is highly sensitive for detecting macular edema, a common complication of diabetic retinopathy characterized by the accumulation of fluid in the macula. OCT allows for quantitative assessment of macular thickness, volume, and morphology, facilitating the diagnosis and monitoring of macular edema over time. Central macular thickness (CMT) measurements obtained by OCT are used as a surrogate marker of disease severity and response to treatment in diabetic macular edema (DME).

2. **Retinal Layer Analysis:** OCT enables segmentation and analysis of individual retinal layers, including the nerve fiber layer (NFL), ganglion cell layer (GCL), inner plexiform layer (IPL), inner nuclear layer (INL), outer plexiform layer (OPL), outer nuclear layer (ONL), photoreceptor layer (PRL), and retinal pigment epithelium (RPE). Quantitative assessment of retinal layer thickness, integrity, and morphology provides insights into the pathophysiology of diabetic retinopathy and the impact of diabetes mellitus on

retinal structure and function.

3. **Identification of Microstructural Abnormalities:** OCT facilitates the identification of microstructural abnormalities associated with diabetic retinopathy, including intraretinal cysts, serous retinal detachment, epiretinal membrane (ERM), vitreomacular traction (VMT), and tractional retinal detachment (TRD). High-resolution OCT imaging allows for visualization of subtle changes in retinal architecture and the presence of tractional forces that contribute to macular distortion and visual impairment in diabetic macular edema (DME) and proliferative diabetic retinopathy (PDR).

4. **Quantitative Analysis of Vascular Changes:** OCT angiography (OCTA) is an extension of OCT that enables non-invasive visualization of retinal and choroidal vasculature by detecting motion contrast of erythrocytes within blood vessels. OCTA provides detailed information about retinal microvasculature, including capillary dropout, microaneurysms, neovascularization, and areas of non-perfusion in diabetic retinopathy. Quantitative analysis of vascular parameters, such as vessel density, perfusion density, and foveal avascular zone (FAZ) metrics, aids in the assessment of disease severity and progression in diabetes mellitus.

## Significance of Optical Coherence Tomography (OCT) in Diabetic Retinopathy:

1. **Early Detection and Diagnosis:** OCT enables the early detection and diagnosis of diabetic retinopathy by providing detailed visualization of retinal morphology and microstructural changes associated with diabetes mellitus. Subtle alterations in retinal thickness, fluid accumulation, and vascular architecture detected by OCT may precede clinically evident signs of diabetic retinopathy on fundoscopic examination, allowing for

early intervention and management to prevent vision loss.

2. **Monitoring of Disease Progression:** OCT facilitates longitudinal monitoring of disease progression and treatment response in diabetic retinopathy by quantifying changes in retinal thickness, morphology, and vascular parameters over time. Serial OCT imaging enables healthcare professionals to assess the efficacy of therapeutic interventions, such as laser photocoagulation, intravitreal injections, or vitrectomy surgery, and modify treatment strategies accordingly to optimize visual outcomes in individuals with diabetes mellitus.

3. **Guidance for Treatment Selection:** OCT findings provide valuable information for guiding treatment selection and personalized management strategies in diabetic retinopathy. Quantitative analysis of macular thickness, edema volume, and retinal layer integrity obtained by OCT aids in risk stratification, prognostication, and decision-making regarding the use of pharmacotherapy, laser therapy, or surgical intervention in diabetic macular edema (DME) and proliferative diabetic retinopathy (PDR).

4. **Patient Education and Counseling:** OCT imaging enhances patient understanding and engagement in the management of diabetic retinopathy by providing visual evidence of retinal pathology and treatment response. Real-time visualization of retinal changes and structural abnormalities on OCT enables healthcare professionals to educate patients about the importance of glycemic control, blood pressure management, and regular ocular screening in the prevention and management of diabetic retinopathy.

In summary, optical coherence tomography (OCT) is a powerful imaging modality for the diagnosis, monitoring, and management of diabetic retinopathy, providing high-resolution, cross-sectional images of retinal morphology, macular edema, and vascular changes associated with diabetes mellitus. OCT enables early detection of diabetic retinopathy, quantitative assessment of disease severity, and guidance for treatment selection, leading to improved visual outcomes and preservation of vision in individuals with diabetes mellitus. Integration of OCT into routine clinical practice enhances patient care, facilitates patient education, and empowers individuals with diabetes to take proactive steps in managing their ocular health.

## Fluorescein Angiography

Fluorescein angiography (FA) is a diagnostic imaging technique used to evaluate retinal vasculature and blood flow dynamics in various ocular diseases, including diabetic retinopathy (DR). It involves the intravenous injection of fluorescein dye, followed by sequential imaging of the retinal circulation using a specialized camera equipped with filters to detect fluorescence. FA provides valuable information about retinal perfusion, capillary leakage, neovascularization, and ischemic areas, aiding in the diagnosis, classification, and management of diabetic retinopathy. This section explores the principles, procedure, clinical applications, and significance of fluorescein angiography in diabetic retinopathy.

### Principles of Fluorescein Angiography:

1. **Fluorescein Dye:** Fluorescein sodium is a water-soluble dye that emits green fluorescence when excited by blue light. It has a high affinity for plasma proteins and binds to albumin in the bloodstream following intravenous injection. Fluorescein dye fluoresces when exposed to specific wavelengths of light, allowing for visualization and imaging of retinal circulation and vascular abnormalities.

2. **Vascular Imaging:** Following intravenous injection, fluorescein dye circulates through the systemic circulation and reaches the retinal vasculature within seconds. The dye traverses retinal arteries, arterioles, capillaries, venules, and veins, providing dynamic visualization of blood flow patterns, perfusion status, and vascular abnormalities in the retina.

3. **Fluorescence Imaging:** A specialized fundus camera equipped with blue excitation light and barrier filters is used to capture sequential images of the retina during fluorescein angiography. The blue excitation light stimulates fluorescein dye, causing it to emit green fluorescence, which is captured by the camera and recorded as digital images or videos. Sequential imaging allows for real-time visualization of dye transit, arteriovenous filling patterns, and late-phase leakage from abnormal retinal vessels.

**Procedure of Fluorescein Angiography:**

1. **Patient Preparation:** Prior to fluorescein angiography, patients are educated about the procedure and potential adverse effects of fluorescein dye, including nausea, vomiting, allergic reactions, and skin discoloration. Consent is obtained, and a thorough medical history is obtained to assess for contraindications, such as allergy to fluorescein dye, pregnancy, and renal impairment.

2. **Intravenous Injection:** A peripheral intravenous catheter is inserted into the antecubital vein, and fluorescein sodium solution (5-10%) is injected rapidly over a few seconds. The dose of fluorescein dye typically ranges from 5 to 5 milliliters, depending on the patient's body weight and renal function. Following injection, the dye rapidly circulates through the bloodstream and reaches the retinal vasculature within seconds.

3. **Image Acquisition:** Sequential imaging of the retina is

performed using a specialized fundus camera equipped with blue excitation light and barrier filters. Images are captured at specific time points, including the early arteriovenous phase (20-30 seconds post-injection), the mid-phase (1-2 minutes post-injection), and the late-phase (5-10 minutes post-injection), to assess dye transit, vascular filling patterns, and leakage from abnormal vessels.

4. **Patient Monitoring:** During fluorescein angiography, patients are closely monitored for adverse reactions, such as nausea, vomiting, dizziness, allergic reactions, and skin discoloration. Visual symptoms, including transient blurring of vision, photophobia, and altered color perception, may occur due to the fluorescent nature of the dye. Prompt management of adverse reactions and supportive care are provided as needed.

**Clinical Applications of Fluorescein Angiography in Diabetic Retinopathy:**

1. **Assessment of Vascular Perfusion:** Fluorescein angiography provides detailed information about retinal perfusion and blood flow dynamics in diabetic retinopathy, including the presence of capillary non-perfusion, arteriovenous shunting, and delayed arteriovenous transit times. Areas of capillary dropout and non-perfusion indicate ischemic retinal zones with an increased risk of neovascularization and vision loss in proliferative diabetic retinopathy (PDR).

2. **Detection of Microaneurysms:** Fluorescein angiography enables the visualization and detection of microaneurysms, small outpouchings of retinal capillaries, which are characteristic early signs of diabetic retinopathy. Microaneurysms appear as hyperfluorescent dots or dots with a halo on fluorescein angiography and indicate localized vascular abnormalities and

microvascular damage in the diabetic retina.

3. **Identification of Leakage Patterns:** Fluorescein angiography allows for the identification and characterization of leakage patterns from abnormal retinal vessels, including microaneurysms, intraretinal hemorrhages, and neovascular tufts. Leakage may manifest as focal, diffuse, or cystoid patterns on fluorescein angiography and correlates with the severity of diabetic macular edema (DME) and the risk of vision loss.

4. **Evaluation of Neovascularization:** Fluorescein angiography plays a crucial role in the detection and classification of neovascularization in diabetic retinopathy, including neovascularization of the optic disc (NVD) and neovascularization elsewhere (NVE). Neovascular tufts and networks appear as hyperfluorescent lesions on fluorescein angiography and indicate pathological angiogenesis and ischemic retinal neovascularization in PDR.

5. **Guidance for Treatment Planning:** Fluorescein angiography provides valuable information for guiding treatment planning and management decisions in diabetic retinopathy. It helps clinicians identify areas of macular ischemia, leakage, and neovascularization that may benefit from laser photocoagulation, intravitreal injections, or surgical intervention to reduce macular edema, inhibit neovascularization, and preserve visual function in individuals with diabetes mellitus.

**Significance of Fluorescein Angiography in Diabetic Retinopathy:**

1. **Early Diagnosis and Classification:** Fluorescein angiography enables the early diagnosis and classification of diabetic retinopathy by visualizing characteristic vascular abnormalities, leakage patterns, and neovascularization associated with diabetes mellitus.

It aids in the differentiation between non-proliferative diabetic retinopathy (NPDR) and proliferative diabetic retinopathy (PDR) and facilitates risk stratification and prognostication in affected individuals.

2. **Monitoring of Disease Progression:** Fluorescein angiography allows for longitudinal monitoring of disease progression and treatment response in diabetic retinopathy by assessing changes in retinal perfusion, vascular leakage, and neovascularization over time. Serial fluorescein angiograms enable clinicians to evaluate the efficacy of therapeutic interventions and modify treatment strategies accordingly to optimize visual outcomes and preserve vision in diabetes mellitus.

3. **Guidance for Treatment Selection:** Fluorescein angiography provides essential information for guiding treatment selection and personalized management strategies in diabetic retinopathy. It helps clinicians identify treatment targets, such as areas of macular edema, ischemia, and neovascularization, and tailor therapeutic interventions, including laser photocoagulation, anti-VEGF therapy, and vitrectomy surgery, to individual patient needs and disease severity.

4. **Research and Clinical Trials:** Fluorescein angiography serves as a valuable tool for research and clinical trials investigating novel therapies and treatment modalities for diabetic retinopathy. It enables researchers to evaluate the efficacy and safety of experimental treatments, assess changes in retinal vasculature and leakage parameters, and elucidate underlying pathophysiological mechanisms contributing to diabetic retinopathy progression.

In summary, fluorescein angiography is a valuable diagnostic imaging technique for evaluating retinal vasculature and blood flow dynamics in diabetic retinopathy, providing essential information for early diagnosis, classification, and management of the disease. It enables clinicians to assess retinal perfusion, detect microvascular abnormalities, characterize leakage patterns, and identify neovascularization associated with diabetes mellitus. Fluorescein angiography plays a crucial role in guiding treatment planning, monitoring disease progression, and optimizing visual outcomes in individuals with diabetic retinopathy, contributing to the preservation of vision and improvement in quality of life in affected patients.

## Retinal Photography

Retinal photography, also known as fundus photography, is a non-invasive imaging technique used to capture high-resolution images of the retina, optic nerve head, and posterior pole of the eye. In the context of diabetic retinopathy (DR), retinal photography plays a crucial role in the screening, diagnosis, monitoring, and documentation of retinal pathology associated with diabetes mellitus. This section provides an overview of retinal photography principles, techniques, clinical applications, and significance in the evaluation of diabetic retinopathy.

### Principles of Retinal Photography:

1. **Imaging Modalities:** Retinal photography utilizes various imaging modalities, including digital fundus cameras, scanning laser ophthalmoscopes (SLOs), and smartphone-based adapters, to capture high-resolution images of the retina. Digital fundus cameras employ a flash or non-mydriatic (non-dilated pupil) imaging system to capture color and red-free fundus images, while SLOs utilize scanning laser technology to acquire multi-modal images, including color, red-free, infrared, and autofluorescence images.

2. **Optical System:** Retinal cameras are equipped with

optical components, such as lenses, filters, and sensors, to optimize image quality, contrast, and resolution. The optical system of a retinal camera focuses light onto the retina and captures reflected or emitted light from retinal structures, including blood vessels, optic disc, macula, and peripheral retina. The quality and clarity of retinal images depend on factors such as camera resolution, sensor sensitivity, and alignment with the patient's pupil.

3. **Field of View:** Retinal photography allows for visualization of different retinal fields, including the central macula, optic disc, posterior pole, and peripheral retina. Wide-field retinal cameras and panoramic imaging techniques enable comprehensive visualization of the entire retina, including the peripheral retina and retinal periphery, facilitating detection of peripheral retinal pathology, such as retinal tears, lattice degeneration, and peripheral neovascularization.

## Techniques of Retinal Photography:

1. **Patient Preparation:** Prior to retinal photography, patients are prepared and positioned for imaging by a trained technician or healthcare professional. Dilating eye drops (mydriatics) may be instilled to dilate the pupil and improve visualization of the retina, particularly in patients with small pupils or media opacities. Proper alignment and fixation are essential for obtaining clear, well-centered retinal images without motion artifacts or blurring.

2. **Image Acquisition:** Retinal images are captured using a digital fundus camera or scanning laser ophthalmoscope (SLO) equipped with a high-resolution sensor and imaging software. The technician adjusts camera settings, such as focus, exposure time, and illumination intensity, to optimize image quality and contrast. Multiple images are acquired from different retinal fields, including the macula, optic disc, and peripheral retina, to provide

comprehensive coverage of the entire retina.

3. **Image Processing:** Retinal images are processed and stored digitally using specialized imaging software, allowing for enhancement, analysis, and interpretation of retinal findings. Image processing techniques, such as contrast adjustment, color balancing, and sharpening, improve image quality and visualization of retinal structures, facilitating accurate diagnosis and documentation of retinal pathology.

## Clinical Applications of Retinal Photography in Diabetic Retinopathy:

1. **Screening and Diagnosis:** Retinal photography is used for screening and diagnosis of diabetic retinopathy by detecting characteristic retinal lesions, including microaneurysms, hemorrhages, exudates, and neovascularization. It enables healthcare professionals to identify early signs of diabetic retinopathy, stratify disease severity, and refer patients for further evaluation and management based on the presence and extent of retinal pathology.

2. **Monitoring and Documentation:** Retinal photography facilitates longitudinal monitoring and documentation of diabetic retinopathy by capturing serial images of retinal changes over time. Serial retinal photographs allow healthcare professionals to track disease progression, assess treatment response, and document retinal findings for clinical decision-making, patient education, and medicolegal purposes.

3. **Telemedicine and Remote Imaging:** Retinal photography enables telemedicine and remote imaging for diabetic retinopathy screening and management, particularly in underserved or remote areas with limited access to ophthalmic specialists. Digital retinal images can be transmitted electronically to remote reading centers or

telemedicine platforms for interpretation and triage, enabling timely diagnosis and intervention for individuals with diabetes mellitus.

4. **Education and Research:** Retinal photography serves as a valuable educational and research tool for studying the pathogenesis, progression, and treatment outcomes of diabetic retinopathy. Retinal images provide visual evidence of retinal pathology and vascular changes associated with diabetes mellitus, facilitating teaching, training, and research endeavors aimed at improving understanding and management of the disease.

## Significance of Retinal Photography in Diabetic Retinopathy:

1. **Early Detection and Intervention:** Retinal photography enables the early detection and intervention of diabetic retinopathy by capturing high-resolution images of retinal lesions and vascular changes associated with diabetes mellitus. Early identification of diabetic retinopathy allows for timely intervention, risk stratification, and implementation of preventive measures to reduce the risk of vision loss and progression to sight-threatening complications.

2. **Longitudinal Monitoring and Management:** Retinal photography facilitates longitudinal monitoring and management of diabetic retinopathy by documenting retinal changes, tracking disease progression, and assessing treatment response over time. Serial retinal images provide valuable insights into the natural history of diabetic retinopathy and the efficacy of therapeutic interventions, guiding personalized management strategies for individuals with diabetes mellitus.

3. **Patient Education and Empowerment:** Retinal photography enhances patient education and empowerment by providing visual evidence of retinal pathology and vascular changes associated with

diabetes mellitus. Retinal images facilitate discussions between healthcare professionals and patients about the importance of glycemic control, blood pressure management, and regular eye examinations in the prevention and management of diabetic retinopathy, empowering individuals with diabetes to take proactive steps in preserving their vision and ocular health.

4. **Resource Optimization and Cost-effectiveness:** Retinal photography contributes to resource optimization and cost-effectiveness in diabetic retinopathy screening and management by streamlining the screening process, reducing the need for dilating eye drops, and enabling telemedicine and remote imaging for underserved populations. Digital retinal images can be stored electronically, shared securely between healthcare providers, and archived for longitudinal follow-up, minimizing the need for repeated imaging and enhancing continuity of care for individuals with diabetes mellitus.

In summary, retinal photography is a valuable diagnostic imaging technique for evaluating retinal pathology and vascular changes associated with diabetic retinopathy. It enables early detection, diagnosis, monitoring, and documentation of diabetic retinopathy by capturing high-resolution images of retinal lesions, tracking disease progression, and assessing treatment response over time. Retinal photography plays a crucial role in screening, management, and education efforts aimed at reducing the burden of diabetic retinopathy and preserving vision in individuals with diabetes mellitus.

# CHAPTER 6: SCREENING AND MONITORING PROTOCOLS

## Recommendations for Screening in Diabetic Patients

Diabetic retinopathy (DR) is a leading cause of vision loss and blindness among individuals with diabetes mellitus (DM). Early detection and timely intervention are crucial for preventing vision-threatening complications and preserving visual function in affected individuals. Screening for diabetic retinopathy aims to identify retinal pathology at an asymptomatic stage, allowing for prompt referral to an eye care specialist and initiation of appropriate management strategies. This section provides an overview of recommendations for screening in diabetic patients, including screening guidelines, risk stratification, screening modalities, and frequency of screening.

## Guidelines and Recommendations:

1. **American Diabetes Association (ADA):** The ADA recommends annual comprehensive eye examinations

for all individuals with type 1 DM and type 2 DM starting at the time of diagnosis. The comprehensive eye examination should include dilated fundus examination (DFE) by an eye care professional, such as an ophthalmologist or optometrist, to assess for the presence of diabetic retinopathy, macular edema, and other ocular complications of diabetes mellitus.

2. **American Academy of Ophthalmology (AAO):** The AAO endorses the ADA guidelines for annual dilated eye examinations in individuals with diabetes mellitus. Additionally, the AAO recommends earlier and more frequent screening for diabetic retinopathy in certain high-risk populations, including individuals with long-standing DM, poor glycemic control, hypertension, nephropathy, and other systemic comorbidities that may increase the risk of retinal vascular complications.

3. **International Council of Ophthalmology (ICO):** The ICO consensus statement on diabetic retinopathy recommends annual or biennial retinal screening for individuals with diabetes mellitus, depending on the level of retinopathy and the presence of risk factors for disease progression. The ICO guidelines emphasize the importance of risk stratification, individualized screening intervals, and timely referral to eye care specialists for further evaluation and management.

## Risk Stratification:

1. **Duration of Diabetes:** Individuals with longer duration of diabetes mellitus are at higher risk of developing diabetic retinopathy and may require more frequent screening intervals. Duration of diabetes is an important risk factor for the development and progression of retinal vascular complications and should be considered in risk stratification and screening recommendations.

2. **Glycemic Control:** Poor glycemic control, as reflected by

elevated hemoglobin A1c (HbA1c) levels, is associated with an increased risk of diabetic retinopathy and progression to sight-threatening complications. Individuals with suboptimal glycemic control may require more frequent retinal screening to detect early signs of retinal pathology and initiate timely intervention to prevent vision loss.

3. **Blood Pressure:** Hypertension is a known risk factor for the development and progression of diabetic retinopathy and other microvascular complications of diabetes mellitus. Individuals with poorly controlled hypertension or evidence of end-organ damage may be at increased risk of retinal vascular complications and may require more frequent retinal screening to monitor for disease progression and optimize blood pressure management.

4. **Renal Function:** Impaired renal function, as evidenced by albuminuria, reduced glomerular filtration rate (GFR), or end-stage renal disease (ESRD), is associated with an increased risk of diabetic retinopathy and progression to proliferative retinopathy and macular edema. Individuals with renal impairment may require more frequent retinal screening and closer monitoring for diabetic retinal complications due to the synergistic effects of diabetes mellitus and renal disease on microvascular function.

## Screening Modalities:

1. **Dilated Fundus Examination (DFE):** Dilated fundus examination by an eye care professional remains the gold standard for diabetic retinopathy screening and evaluation. DFE allows for direct visualization of the retina, optic nerve head, and macula to assess for the presence of retinal lesions, microaneurysms, hemorrhages, exudates, and neovascularization associated with diabetic retinopathy.

2. **Digital Retinal Photography:** Digital retinal photography or fundus imaging is a non-invasive imaging

modality used for diabetic retinopathy screening and documentation. It involves capturing high-resolution color fundus images of the retina using a digital fundus camera or smartphone-based adapter. Retinal photographs are evaluated by trained graders or interpreted using automated image analysis software to detect retinal pathology and stratify disease severity.

3. **Optical Coherence Tomography (OCT):** Optical coherence tomography (OCT) is a high-resolution imaging technique used to assess retinal thickness, morphology, and macular edema in diabetic retinopathy. OCT enables visualization of retinal layers, measurement of central macular thickness (CMT), and detection of intraretinal cysts, subretinal fluid, and epiretinal membranes associated with diabetic macular edema (DME).

4. **Fluorescein Angiography (FA):** Fluorescein angiography is an invasive imaging technique used for the evaluation of retinal vasculature, perfusion, and leakage patterns in diabetic retinopathy. FA involves the intravenous injection of fluorescein dye, followed by sequential imaging of retinal circulation using a specialized fundus camera equipped with blue excitation light and barrier filters.

**Frequency of Screening:**

1. **Annual Screening:** Annual dilated eye examinations are recommended for all individuals with diabetes mellitus, starting at the time of diagnosis, to screen for diabetic retinopathy and other ocular complications of diabetes. Annual screening allows for early detection of retinal pathology, timely referral to eye care specialists, and implementation of preventive measures to reduce the risk of vision loss in affected individuals.

2. **Biennial Screening:** Biennial retinal screening may be considered for individuals with well-controlled type 2 diabetes mellitus, no evidence of retinopathy on previous

examinations, and no other significant risk factors for diabetic retinopathy progression. Biennial screening intervals should be individualized based on the patient's age, duration of diabetes, glycemic control, blood pressure, and other systemic comorbidities.

3. **More Frequent Screening:** Individuals with high-risk features for diabetic retinopathy, such as longer duration of diabetes, poor glycemic control, hypertension, nephropathy, or other systemic comorbidities, may require more frequent retinal screening intervals. More frequent screening intervals should be tailored to individual patient needs and risk factors to optimize detection of retinal pathology and prevent vision loss in high-risk populations.

4. **Individualized Screening:** Screening intervals for diabetic retinopathy should be individualized based on the patient's age, duration of diabetes, glycemic control, blood pressure, renal function, and other systemic comorbidities. Individualized screening recommendations should take into account the patient's overall health status, life expectancy, preferences, and access to eye care services to optimize the delivery of diabetic retinopathy screening and management.

In summary, recommendations for screening in diabetic patients emphasize the importance of annual dilated eye examinations for early detection and timely intervention of diabetic retinopathy. Screening guidelines recommend risk stratification, individualized screening intervals, and the use of multiple screening modalities, including dilated fundus examination, digital retinal photography, optical coherence tomography, and fluorescein angiography, to optimize detection of retinal pathology and preserve visual function in individuals with diabetes mellitus. Implementation of screening programs, patient education, and interdisciplinary collaboration among healthcare professionals are essential for reducing the burden of diabetic retinopathy and improving eye care outcomes in diabetic patients.

## Frequency of Screening Examinations

Determining the appropriate frequency of screening examinations for diabetic retinopathy (DR) is crucial in optimizing early detection and management of retinal pathology while minimizing unnecessary healthcare utilization. The frequency of screening examinations depends on various factors, including the individual's risk profile, type of diabetes, duration of disease, glycemic control, and presence of systemic comorbidities. This section provides an overview of the recommended frequency of screening examinations for diabetic retinopathy based on current guidelines and risk stratification.

### Annual Screening:

1. **Type 1 Diabetes Mellitus (T1DM):** Individuals with type 1 diabetes mellitus are at increased risk of developing diabetic retinopathy, particularly with longer disease duration. Therefore, annual dilated eye examinations are recommended for all individuals with type 1 diabetes, beginning within five years after the onset of diabetes diagnosis, regardless of age.

2. **Type 2 Diabetes Mellitus (T2DM):** Annual dilated eye examinations are also recommended for individuals with type 2 diabetes mellitus, starting at the time of diabetes diagnosis. However, in cases of newly diagnosed type 2 diabetes with no evidence of retinopathy, screening can be deferred until the patient has had diabetes for five years.

### High-Risk Groups:

1. **High-Risk Features:** Individuals with high-risk features

for diabetic retinopathy, such as poor glycemic control (HbA1c > 7%), hypertension, nephropathy, or pregnancy, may require more frequent screening examinations. In such cases, annual or even more frequent screening intervals may be warranted to detect and manage retinal pathology promptly.

2. **Pregnancy:** Pregnant individuals with pre-existing diabetes or gestational diabetes mellitus (GDM) are at increased risk of developing diabetic retinopathy or exacerbating pre-existing retinopathy due to hormonal changes and metabolic fluctuations during pregnancy. Therefore, pregnant women with diabetes should undergo dilated eye examinations before conception and during each trimester of pregnancy to monitor for retinal changes and prevent vision loss.

## Biennial Screening:

1. **Stable, Low-Risk Patients:** Individuals with well-controlled type 2 diabetes mellitus, no evidence of diabetic retinopathy on previous examinations, and no other significant risk factors for disease progression may undergo biennial dilated eye examinations. Biennial screening intervals should be individualized based on the patient's age, duration of diabetes, glycemic control, blood pressure, and overall health status.

2. **Telemedicine Screening:** In select cases, telemedicine-based diabetic retinopathy screening programs may use digital retinal photography or teleophthalmology to provide remote retinal evaluations for individuals with diabetes mellitus. Telemedicine screening may be particularly beneficial for underserved populations, remote areas, or individuals with limited access to eye care services.

## Individualized Screening:

1. **Clinical Judgment:** The frequency of screening examinations for diabetic retinopathy should be individualized based on the patient's risk profile, medical history, visual status, and preferences. Healthcare providers should use clinical judgment and evidence-based guidelines to determine the appropriate screening intervals for each patient, considering factors such as age, duration of diabetes, glycemic control, blood pressure, renal function, and presence of systemic comorbidities.

2. **Shared Decision-Making:** Shared decision-making between healthcare providers and patients is essential in establishing personalized screening schedules for diabetic retinopathy. Patients should be educated about the importance of regular eye examinations, the risks of diabetic retinopathy, and the benefits of early detection and intervention in preserving visual function.

**Longitudinal Monitoring:**

1. **Serial Imaging:** Serial retinal imaging, such as digital fundus photography or optical coherence tomography (OCT), may be utilized for longitudinal monitoring of diabetic retinopathy progression and treatment response over time. Serial imaging allows healthcare providers to track changes in retinal pathology, assess disease severity, and adjust management strategies accordingly.

2. **Integrated Care:** Integrated care models that incorporate diabetic retinopathy screening into primary care settings or diabetes management programs can improve access to eye care services, enhance patient engagement, and facilitate timely detection and management of retinal pathology in individuals with diabetes mellitus.

In summary, the frequency of screening examinations for diabetic retinopathy should be tailored to the individual patient's risk profile, type of diabetes, duration of disease, glycemic control, and presence of systemic comorbidities. Annual dilated eye examinations are recommended for all individuals with diabetes mellitus, with consideration of more frequent screening intervals for high-risk groups and pregnant individuals. Biennial screening may be appropriate for stable, low-risk patients, while telemedicine screening and shared decision-making can enhance access to eye care services and optimize early detection and management of diabetic retinopathy. Longitudinal monitoring through serial retinal imaging and integrated care models can further support comprehensive diabetic retinopathy screening and management efforts, leading to improved visual outcomes and preservation of vision in affected individuals.

## Importance of Early Detection and Intervention

Early detection and intervention are paramount in the management of diabetic retinopathy (DR) to prevent vision loss and preserve visual function in individuals with diabetes mellitus (DM). Diabetic retinopathy is a progressive microvascular complication of DM characterized by retinal vascular changes, including microaneurysms, hemorrhages, exudates, and neovascularization, which can lead to macular edema, retinal detachment, and vision-threatening complications if left untreated. This section explores the significance of early detection and intervention in diabetic retinopathy and its impact on visual outcomes and quality of life.

### Prevention of Vision Loss:

1. **Preservation of Visual Function:** Early detection of diabetic retinopathy allows for prompt initiation of preventive measures and therapeutic interventions to preserve visual function and prevent irreversible vision

loss. Timely intervention can mitigate the progression of retinal pathology, reduce the risk of sight-threatening complications, and optimize visual outcomes in affected individuals.

2. **Treatment of Macular Edema:** Diabetic macular edema (DME) is a common complication of diabetic retinopathy characterized by the accumulation of fluid within the macula, leading to central vision loss and impairment of visual acuity. Early detection of DME through comprehensive eye examinations and retinal imaging enables timely initiation of treatment modalities, such as anti-vascular endothelial growth factor (anti-VEGF) injections, intravitreal corticosteroids, or laser photocoagulation, to reduce macular edema, improve visual acuity, and prevent further vision loss.

3. **Prevention of Proliferative Disease:** Proliferative diabetic retinopathy (PDR) is an advanced stage of diabetic retinopathy characterized by the growth of abnormal blood vessels on the retina and optic disc, leading to vitreous hemorrhage, retinal detachment, and neovascular glaucoma. Early detection and treatment of non-proliferative diabetic retinopathy (NPDR) can prevent the progression to PDR by addressing underlying retinal ischemia, reducing vascular leakage, and inhibiting neovascularization.

## Optimization of Treatment Outcomes:

1. **Maximization of Visual Potential:** Early detection of diabetic retinopathy allows for timely implementation of therapeutic interventions aimed at maximizing visual potential and preserving quality of life in affected individuals. Early treatment of macular edema, proliferative disease, and other retinal complications can help maintain functional vision, enhance visual acuity, and improve patients' ability to perform daily activities

and tasks.

2. **Minimization of Disease Progression:** Early intervention in diabetic retinopathy can minimize the progression of retinal pathology, reduce the need for invasive procedures, and prevent irreversible vision loss in affected individuals. By addressing modifiable risk factors, such as hyperglycemia, hypertension, dyslipidemia, and smoking, healthcare providers can mitigate the systemic and ocular manifestations of diabetes mellitus and optimize treatment outcomes in diabetic retinopathy.

3. **Prevention of Complications:** Early detection and intervention in diabetic retinopathy can prevent the development of vision-threatening complications, such as vitreous hemorrhage, tractional retinal detachment, and neovascular glaucoma, which may require surgical intervention and may result in permanent visual impairment or blindness if left untreated. By addressing retinal pathology at an early stage, healthcare providers can minimize the risk of complications and improve long-term visual prognosis in individuals with diabetes mellitus.

## Patient Education and Empowerment:

1. **Awareness of Eye Health:** Early detection of diabetic retinopathy emphasizes the importance of regular eye examinations, adherence to treatment regimens, and proactive management of diabetes mellitus to preserve vision and ocular health. Patient education and empowerment play a crucial role in raising awareness of eye health, promoting self-management behaviors, and encouraging individuals with diabetes to prioritize regular eye care as part of their overall diabetes management plan.

2. **Engagement in Care:** Early intervention in diabetic retinopathy fosters patient engagement and participation in eye care services, enabling individuals with diabetes

mellitus to take an active role in monitoring their ocular health, adhering to treatment recommendations, and making informed decisions about their visual care. By empowering patients with knowledge and resources, healthcare providers can enhance patient engagement, improve treatment adherence, and optimize treatment outcomes in diabetic retinopathy.

**Healthcare System Benefits:**

1. **Cost Savings:** Early detection and intervention in diabetic retinopathy result in cost savings for healthcare systems by reducing the burden of vision loss, preventing expensive surgical interventions, and minimizing the economic impact of disability and productivity loss associated with visual impairment. By investing in preventive eye care and early treatment modalities, healthcare systems can achieve long-term cost savings and improve the efficiency of healthcare delivery for individuals with diabetes mellitus.

2. **Resource Allocation:** Early detection and intervention in diabetic retinopathy optimize resource allocation and healthcare utilization by targeting high-risk individuals, implementing evidence-based screening protocols, and prioritizing interventions based on disease severity and progression. By allocating resources strategically to preventive care, screening programs, and treatment services, healthcare systems can improve access to eye care services, reduce disparities in visual health outcomes, and enhance the overall efficiency of healthcare delivery for diabetic patients.

In summary, early detection and intervention are essential in the management of diabetic retinopathy to prevent vision loss, preserve visual function, and optimize treatment outcomes in individuals with diabetes mellitus. By emphasizing the importance of regular eye examinations, proactive management of diabetes mellitus, and patient engagement in eye care services, healthcare providers can promote awareness of eye health, empower patients to prioritize ocular health, and achieve long-term improvements in visual outcomes and quality of life for individuals affected by diabetic retinopathy. Through collaborative efforts among healthcare providers, patients, and healthcare systems, early detection and intervention can mitigate the progression of diabetic retinopathy, reduce the burden of visual impairment, and promote lifelong ocular health in diabetic patients.

# CHAPTER 7: MANAGEMENT STRATEGIES

## Lifestyle Modifications and Glycemic Control

Effective management of diabetic retinopathy (DR) requires a comprehensive approach that includes lifestyle modifications aimed at optimizing glycemic control. Lifestyle interventions play a crucial role in reducing the risk of retinal complications, slowing disease progression, and preserving visual function in individuals with diabetes mellitus (DM). This section discusses the importance of lifestyle modifications and strategies for achieving glycemic control to prevent and manage diabetic retinopathy.

## Importance of Lifestyle Modifications:

1 **Role in Disease Prevention:** Lifestyle modifications, including dietary changes, physical activity, weight management, and smoking cessation, are essential for preventing the development of diabetic retinopathy and other microvascular complications in individuals at risk of diabetes mellitus. Adopting a healthy lifestyle can improve insulin sensitivity, reduce systemic inflammation, and minimize oxidative stress, thereby mitigating

the underlying pathophysiological mechanisms contributing to diabetic retinopathy progression.

2 **Impact on Disease Progression:** Lifestyle modifications can slow the progression of diabetic retinopathy by addressing modifiable risk factors, such as hyperglycemia, hypertension, dyslipidemia, and obesity, which contribute to retinal vascular damage and macular edema. By promoting glycemic control and cardiovascular health, lifestyle interventions can reduce the risk of sight-threatening complications, such as proliferative diabetic retinopathy (PDR) and diabetic macular edema (DME), and improve long-term visual outcomes in individuals with diabetes mellitus.

3 **Enhancement of Treatment Efficacy:** Lifestyle modifications can enhance the efficacy of pharmacological and surgical interventions for diabetic retinopathy by optimizing metabolic parameters, promoting tissue healing, and improving treatment response. Adherence to a healthy lifestyle can complement medical therapy, laser photocoagulation, intravitreal injections, and vitreoretinal surgery in the management of diabetic retinopathy, leading to better treatment outcomes and preservation of visual function.

**Dietary Modifications:**

1 **Glycemic Control:** Dietary modifications play a central role in glycemic control and diabetes management, influencing blood glucose levels, insulin sensitivity, and postprandial glycemic excursions. Individuals with diabetes mellitus should adhere to a balanced diet that includes complex carbohydrates, fiber-rich foods, lean proteins, and healthy fats to minimize glycemic variability and optimize metabolic control. Carbohydrate counting, glycemic index/load considerations, and portion control are important dietary strategies for managing blood glucose levels and preventing hyperglycemia-related retinal damage.

2 **Nutritional Supplements:** Certain nutritional supplements, such as omega-3 fatty acids, antioxidants (e.g., vitamins C and E, zinc), and lutein/zeaxanthin, may have potential benefits in the prevention and management of diabetic retinopathy by reducing oxidative stress, inflammation, and lipid peroxidation in the retina. However, the evidence regarding the efficacy of nutritional supplements in diabetic retinopathy is still evolving, and supplementation should be individualized based on the patient's nutritional status, dietary intake, and risk profile.

### Physical Activity:

1 **Impact on Insulin Sensitivity:** Regular physical activity improves insulin sensitivity, glucose uptake, and glycemic control in individuals with diabetes mellitus, leading to reduced blood glucose levels and decreased risk of microvascular complications, including diabetic retinopathy. Aerobic exercise, resistance training, and flexibility exercises are recommended components of a comprehensive exercise regimen for individuals with diabetes, aiming to achieve at least 150 minutes of moderate-intensity aerobic activity per week, supplemented with muscle-strengthening activities on two or more days per week.

2 **Cardiovascular Benefits:** Physical activity provides additional cardiovascular benefits beyond glycemic control, including reduction of blood pressure, improvement of lipid profile, enhancement of endothelial function, and promotion of weight loss, which are important considerations in the management of diabetic retinopathy risk factors and comorbidities. Regular exercise can attenuate systemic inflammation, oxidative stress, and vascular dysfunction associated with diabetes mellitus, contributing to the prevention and management of retinal vascular complications.

### Weight Management:

1 **Obesity and Diabetes:** Obesity is a major risk factor for the development and progression of diabetic retinopathy, as it exacerbates insulin resistance, dyslipidemia, and systemic inflammation, which contribute to retinal vascular dysfunction and macular edema. Weight management strategies, including calorie restriction, portion control, and dietary modifications, are essential for achieving and maintaining optimal body weight in individuals with diabetes mellitus, thereby reducing the risk of diabetic retinopathy and improving metabolic control.

2 **Bariatric Surgery:** Bariatric surgery may be considered in severely obese individuals with type 2 diabetes mellitus who have not achieved adequate glycemic control with lifestyle modifications and medical therapy. Bariatric surgery can lead to significant weight loss, improvement in insulin sensitivity, resolution of diabetes mellitus, and reduction in cardiovascular risk factors, which may have beneficial effects on diabetic retinopathy progression and visual outcomes in select patients.

**Smoking Cessation:**

1 **Impact on Vascular Health:** Smoking is a well-established risk factor for the development and progression of diabetic retinopathy, as it promotes vascular endothelial dysfunction, oxidative stress, and microvascular damage in the retina. Smoking cessation is essential for preserving visual function and preventing sight-threatening complications in individuals with diabetes mellitus, as it reduces the risk of retinal vascular leakage, neovascularization, and progression to proliferative disease.

2 **Multifaceted Approach:** Smoking cessation interventions should involve a multifaceted approach, including behavioral counseling, pharmacotherapy (e.g., nicotine replacement therapy, bupropion, varenicline), and supportive resources to address nicotine dependence, withdrawal symptoms, and psychosocial factors associated with smoking cessation. Healthcare providers

play a pivotal role in promoting smoking cessation and providing personalized support to individuals with diabetes mellitus who smoke, emphasizing the importance of quitting for overall health and ocular well-being.

## Glycemic Control:

1 **Hemoglobin A1c (HbA1c) Targets:** Glycemic control is a cornerstone of diabetes management and a key determinant of retinal health in individuals with diabetes mellitus. The American Diabetes Association (ADA) recommends individualized glycemic targets based on age, life expectancy, comorbidities, and patient preferences, with a general goal of achieving an HbA1c level <7% in most adults with diabetes mellitus to reduce the risk of microvascular complications, including diabetic retinopathy.

2 **Glucose Monitoring:** Regular self-monitoring of blood glucose levels is essential for optimizing glycemic control and preventing hyperglycemia-related retinal damage in individuals with diabetes mellitus. Blood glucose monitoring allows patients to assess their response to dietary modifications, physical activity, medication regimens, and lifestyle changes, empowering them to make informed decisions about their diabetes management and adjust their treatment strategies as needed to achieve target glycemic levels.

## Conclusion:

Lifestyle modifications, including dietary changes, physical activity, weight management, and smoking cessation, are integral components of diabetic retinopathy management and glycemic control in individuals with diabetes mellitus. By addressing modifiable risk factors and promoting healthy behaviors, healthcare providers can empower patients to take an active role in managing their diabetes and reducing the risk of retinal complications. A multidisciplinary approach that integrates lifestyle interventions with medical therapy, retinal screening, and ophthalmic care is essential for optimizing visual outcomes and preserving ocular health in individuals affected by diabetic retinopathy. Through collaborative efforts among healthcare providers, patients, and community resources, lifestyle modifications can play a pivotal role in preventing, delaying, and mitigating the progression of diabetic retinopathy, ultimately improving the quality of life and visual prognosis for individuals with diabetes mellitus.

## Pharmacological Interventions: Anti-VEGF Therapy and Corticosteroids

Pharmacological interventions play a crucial role in the management of diabetic retinopathy (DR) by targeting key pathophysiological mechanisms underlying retinal vascular dysfunction, macular edema, and neovascularization. Anti-vascular endothelial growth factor (anti-VEGF) agents and corticosteroids are the mainstay of pharmacotherapy for diabetic macular edema (DME) and proliferative diabetic retinopathy (PDR), offering effective treatment options to preserve visual function and prevent vision loss in individuals with diabetes mellitus (DM). This section provides an overview of anti-VEGF therapy, corticosteroids, and their role in the management of diabetic retinopathy.

### Anti-VEGF Therapy:

1 **Mechanism of Action:** Anti-VEGF therapy targets vascular endothelial growth factor (VEGF), a key mediator of angiogenesis, vascular permeability, and inflammation in diabetic retinopathy. VEGF promotes neovascularization, vascular leakage, and retinal edema by stimulating endothelial cell proliferation, migration, and vascular permeability, contributing to the development and

progression of diabetic macular edema (DME) and proliferative diabetic retinopathy (PDR). Anti-VEGF agents block the activity of VEGF, inhibiting neovascularization, reducing vascular permeability, and improving macular edema in individuals with diabetic retinopathy.

2 **Intravitreal Injections:** Anti-VEGF agents, including ranibizumab, aflibercept, and bevacizumab, are administered via intravitreal injections into the vitreous cavity, allowing for targeted delivery of therapeutic agents to the retina and macula. Intravitreal injections provide sustained therapeutic concentrations of anti-VEGF agents within the eye, minimizing systemic exposure and maximizing local efficacy in treating diabetic macular edema and proliferative diabetic retinopathy.

3 **Efficacy in Diabetic Macular Edema:** Anti-VEGF therapy has demonstrated significant efficacy in the treatment of diabetic macular edema, leading to improvements in visual acuity, reduction of central macular thickness, and stabilization of retinal function in clinical trials and real-world studies. Anti-VEGF agents are considered first-line treatments for center-involved DME, offering superior efficacy compared to laser photocoagulation and corticosteroid therapy in improving visual outcomes and reducing the risk of vision loss.

4 **Efficacy in Proliferative Disease:** Anti-VEGF therapy has also shown promise in the management of proliferative diabetic retinopathy, particularly as an adjunctive treatment to panretinal photocoagulation (PRP) laser therapy. Anti-VEGF agents can induce regression of neovascularization, reduce the need for additional laser treatments, and improve the safety profile of PRP by minimizing the risk of visual field loss, macular edema, and other complications associated with traditional laser therapy alone.

5 **Treatment Regimens:** Anti-VEGF therapy is typically administered using a proactive or reactive treatment regimen,

depending on the severity of diabetic retinopathy, the presence of macular edema, and the individual patient's response to therapy. Proactive treatment involves regular monitoring and scheduled intravitreal injections of anti-VEGF agents based on predefined intervals, while reactive treatment involves initiation of therapy in response to worsening retinal pathology or visual decline.

## Corticosteroids:

1 **Mechanism of Action:** Corticosteroids exert anti-inflammatory, anti-edematous, and anti-angiogenic effects in diabetic retinopathy by suppressing the production of pro-inflammatory cytokines, inhibiting leukocyte activation, and stabilizing vascular endothelial barriers. Corticosteroids also modulate the expression of VEGF, interleukins, and other mediators of inflammation and angiogenesis implicated in the pathogenesis of diabetic macular edema and proliferative retinopathy.

2 **Intravitreal Implants:** Corticosteroids are administered via intravitreal implants or injections into the vitreous cavity, allowing for sustained release of therapeutic agents to the retina and macula over an extended period. Intravitreal corticosteroid implants, such as dexamethasone intravitreal implant (DEX implant) and fluocinolone acetonide intravitreal implant (FA implant), provide localized delivery of corticosteroids, minimizing systemic side effects and maximizing ocular efficacy in treating diabetic retinopathy.

3 **Efficacy in Diabetic Macular Edema:** Intravitreal corticosteroids have demonstrated efficacy in the treatment of diabetic macular edema, leading to improvements in visual acuity, reduction of macular thickness, and resolution of retinal edema in clinical trials and real-world studies. Corticosteroid implants offer sustained release of therapeutic agents, allowing for less frequent dosing compared to intravitreal injections and providing long-term control of macular edema in individuals with diabetes mellitus.

4 **Efficacy in Proliferative Disease:** Corticosteroids may also be beneficial in the management of proliferative diabetic retinopathy, particularly in cases of vitreous hemorrhage, tractional retinal detachment, or refractory neovascularization. Intravitreal corticosteroid therapy can stabilize retinal neovascularization, reduce fibrovascular proliferation, and promote regression of abnormal blood vessels, complementing panretinal photocoagulation (PRP) laser therapy in the treatment of proliferative retinopathy.

5 **Safety Considerations:** Despite their efficacy, corticosteroids are associated with potential ocular and systemic side effects, including cataract formation, intraocular pressure elevation, glaucoma, and exacerbation of systemic comorbidities. Patient selection, monitoring, and individualized treatment regimens are essential considerations in the use of intravitreal corticosteroids for diabetic retinopathy to minimize the risk of adverse events and optimize treatment outcomes.

## Conclusion:

Anti-VEGF therapy and corticosteroids are effective pharmacological interventions for the management of diabetic retinopathy, offering targeted approaches to reduce retinal vascular leakage, macular edema, and neovascularization in individuals with diabetes mellitus. These treatments play a pivotal role in preserving visual function, preventing vision loss, and improving quality of life in patients with diabetic retinopathy, particularly those with center-involved diabetic macular edema and proliferative disease. By addressing underlying pathophysiological mechanisms and modifiable risk factors, anti-VEGF therapy and corticosteroids complement traditional laser photocoagulation and surgical interventions, providing additional treatment options to optimize visual outcomes and enhance long-term ocular health in individuals affected by diabetic retinopathy. Through evidence-based practice, patient-centered care, and interdisciplinary collaboration among ophthalmologists, retina specialists, endocrinologists, and primary care providers, pharmacological interventions can play a pivotal role in the holistic management of diabetic retinopathy and the prevention of vision loss in individuals with diabetes mellitus.

## Laser Therapy: Panretinal Photocoagulation and Focal Laser Treatment

Laser therapy is a cornerstone of treatment for diabetic retinopathy (DR), offering targeted photocoagulation to address specific retinal lesions and pathologies associated with the disease. Panretinal photocoagulation (PRP) and focal laser treatment are two main modalities used in the management of DR, each serving distinct purposes in the preservation of visual function and prevention of vision loss in individuals with diabetes mellitus (DM). This section provides an overview of PRP and focal laser treatment and their roles in the management of diabetic retinopathy.

### Panretinal Photocoagulation (PRP):

1 **Mechanism of Action:** Panretinal photocoagulation (PRP) involves the application of laser burns to the peripheral retina, targeting ischemic areas and promoting regression of abnormal blood vessels, neovascularization, and fibrovascular proliferation characteristic of proliferative diabetic retinopathy (PDR). PRP induces photocoagulation of the retinal tissue, reducing oxygen demand, improving retinal perfusion, and inhibiting the release of angiogenic factors, such as vascular endothelial growth factor (VEGF), which contribute to the pathogenesis of neovascularization.

2 **Indications:** PRP is indicated for the treatment of proliferative diabetic retinopathy (PDR) and high-risk characteristics, such as neovascularization of the optic disc (NVD) and neovascularization elsewhere (NVE), which pose a significant risk of vision loss due to vitreous hemorrhage, tractional retinal detachment, and neovascular glaucoma. PRP aims to reduce the risk of vision-threatening complications by inducing regression of abnormal blood vessels, stabilizing retinal neovascularization, and preventing disease progression in individuals with diabetes mellitus.

3 **Treatment Protocol:** PRP is typically performed using a laser photocoagulator equipped with a slit lamp delivery system or a laser indirect ophthalmoscope, allowing for precise application of laser burns to the peripheral retina. Multiple laser sessions may be required to achieve adequate panretinal coverage and regression of neovascularization, with treatment endpoints based on the extent of retinal ischemia, the presence of new vessels, and the risk of vision loss in individual patients.

4 **Efficacy:** PRP has been shown to be effective in reducing the risk of severe visual loss and preventing vision-threatening complications in individuals with proliferative diabetic retinopathy. Clinical trials and real-world studies have demonstrated the efficacy of PRP in stabilizing retinal neovascularization, reducing the incidence of vitreous hemorrhage and tractional retinal detachment, and preserving visual function in patients with diabetes mellitus. Early intervention with PRP can prevent disease progression and optimize long-term visual outcomes in individuals with proliferative disease.

**Focal Laser Treatment:**

1 **Mechanism of Action:** Focal laser treatment involves the application of laser burns to discrete retinal lesions, such as

microaneurysms, intraretinal hemorrhages, and focal areas of leakage, characteristic of diabetic macular edema (DME) and clinically significant macular edema (CSME). Focal laser treatment aims to reduce macular edema, stabilize retinal architecture, and improve visual acuity by sealing leaking microaneurysms, reducing vascular permeability, and promoting resolution of intraretinal fluid accumulation in the macula.

2 **Indications:** Focal laser treatment is indicated for the management of diabetic macular edema (DME) and clinically significant macular edema (CSME), particularly in cases of center-involved DME with retinal thickening involving or threatening the fovea. Focal laser treatment aims to improve central vision, reduce the risk of vision loss, and enhance visual function by addressing the underlying macular pathology and minimizing the impact of macular edema on retinal function in individuals with diabetes mellitus.

3 **Treatment Protocol:** Focal laser treatment is typically performed using a laser photocoagulator equipped with a slit lamp delivery system or a fundus contact lens, allowing for precise targeting of laser burns to the macular region. Laser burns are applied in a grid pattern or around focal leakage sites identified on fluorescein angiography, aiming to reduce macular edema, promote macular remodeling, and improve visual outcomes in patients with diabetic retinopathy.

4 **Efficacy:** Focal laser treatment has been shown to be effective in reducing macular edema, stabilizing visual acuity, and improving retinal function in individuals with diabetic macular edema (DME) and clinically significant macular edema (CSME). Clinical trials and real-world studies have demonstrated the efficacy of focal laser treatment in reducing central macular thickness, improving visual acuity, and minimizing the risk of vision loss in patients with diabetes mellitus. Early intervention with focal laser treatment can prevent progression of macular edema and

optimize long-term visual outcomes in individuals with diabetic retinopathy.

### Conclusion:

Panretinal photocoagulation (PRP) and focal laser treatment are essential modalities in the management of diabetic retinopathy, offering targeted approaches to reduce retinal ischemia, neovascularization, and macular edema in individuals with diabetes mellitus. PRP aims to prevent vision-threatening complications associated with proliferative diabetic retinopathy (PDR), while focal laser treatment targets macular edema and preserves central vision in diabetic macular edema (DME). By addressing specific retinal pathologies and risk factors for vision loss, laser therapy plays a pivotal role in preserving visual function, preventing blindness, and optimizing long-term ocular health outcomes in patients with diabetic retinopathy. Through evidence-based practice, individualized treatment planning, and interdisciplinary collaboration among ophthalmologists, retina specialists, and diabetes care providers, laser therapy can complement pharmacological interventions, surgical procedures, and lifestyle modifications in the holistic management of diabetic retinopathy, ultimately improving visual outcomes and quality of life for individuals affected by diabetes mellitus.

### Surgical Interventions: Vitrectomy and Retinal Detachment Repair

Surgical interventions play a crucial role in the management of advanced diabetic retinopathy (DR) and its complications, including vitreous hemorrhage, tractional retinal detachment, and proliferative vitreoretinopathy (PVR). Vitrectomy and retinal detachment repair are two main surgical procedures used in the treatment of diabetic retinopathy, aiming to restore retinal anatomy, preserve visual function, and prevent irreversible vision loss in individuals with diabetes mellitus (DM). This section provides an overview of vitrectomy and retinal detachment repair and their roles in the surgical management of diabetic retinopathy.

**Vitrectomy:**

1 **Indications:** Vitrectomy is indicated for the treatment of complications associated with proliferative diabetic retinopathy (PDR), including non-clearing vitreous hemorrhage, tractional retinal detachment, epiretinal membrane formation, and diabetic macular traction syndrome. Vitrectomy aims to remove vitreous opacities, release tractional forces on the retina, and restore retinal anatomy, thereby improving visual function and preventing further progression of diabetic retinopathy in individuals with diabetes mellitus.

2 **Surgical Technique:** Vitrectomy involves the removal of the vitreous gel from the posterior segment of the eye using microsurgical instrumentation, including vitreous cutters, infusion cannulas, and light sources, under direct visualization through a microscope or wide-angle viewing system. The surgical procedure may be combined with membrane peeling, endolaser photocoagulation, and intraocular tamponade with gas or silicone oil to address associated retinal pathologies, such as epiretinal membranes, fibrovascular proliferation, and retinal tears.

3 **Outcomes:** Vitrectomy has been shown to be effective in improving visual acuity, resolving vitreous hemorrhage, flattening retinal detachments, and stabilizing retinal function in individuals with proliferative diabetic retinopathy. Clinical studies and real-world evidence have demonstrated favorable outcomes with vitrectomy in terms of visual recovery, anatomic success, and prevention of recurrent complications in patients

with diabetes mellitus. Early intervention with vitrectomy can prevent progression to severe vision loss and enhance long-term visual outcomes in individuals with advanced diabetic retinopathy.

**Retinal Detachment Repair:**

1 **Indications:** Retinal detachment repair is indicated for the management of tractional retinal detachment, rhegmatogenous retinal detachment, and combined tractional-rhegmatogenous detachments associated with proliferative diabetic retinopathy (PDR) and tractional diabetic macular edema (DME). Retinal detachment repair aims to reattach the detached retina, seal retinal breaks, and restore retinal function, thereby preserving visual acuity and preventing permanent vision loss in individuals with diabetes mellitus.

2 **Surgical Techniques:** Retinal detachment repair may involve a combination of scleral buckling, pars plana vitrectomy, pneumatic retinopexy, and silicone oil or gas tamponade to achieve retinal reattachment and stabilize the retina. Scleral buckling involves the placement of a silicone band around the sclera to indent the eyeball and support the detached retina, while vitrectomy allows for removal of vitreous traction, drainage of subretinal fluid, and endolaser photocoagulation to seal retinal breaks and prevent recurrence of detachment.

3 **Outcomes:** Retinal detachment repair has demonstrated favorable outcomes in terms of anatomical success, visual recovery, and prevention of recurrent detachment in individuals with proliferative diabetic retinopathy and tractional retinal detachments. Clinical studies and surgical series have reported high rates of retinal reattachment, stabilization of visual acuity, and long-term maintenance of retinal function following retinal detachment repair in patients with diabetes mellitus. Timely intervention with retinal detachment repair can prevent irreversible vision loss and optimize visual outcomes in

individuals with advanced diabetic retinopathy.

## Conclusion:

Vitrectomy and retinal detachment repair are essential surgical interventions in the management of advanced diabetic retinopathy and its complications, offering effective strategies to restore retinal anatomy, preserve visual function, and prevent irreversible vision loss in individuals with diabetes mellitus. These surgical procedures play a pivotal role in addressing vitreoretinal pathology, such as vitreous hemorrhage, tractional retinal detachment, and proliferative vitreoretinopathy, which can lead to severe vision loss if left untreated. Through interdisciplinary collaboration among vitreoretinal surgeons, ophthalmologists, and diabetes care providers, surgical interventions can complement pharmacological therapies, laser treatments, and lifestyle modifications in the holistic management of diabetic retinopathy, ultimately improving visual outcomes and quality of life for individuals affected by diabetes mellitus. By addressing sight-threatening complications and preserving ocular health, vitrectomy and retinal detachment repair contribute to the prevention of blindness and the promotion of lifelong ocular wellness in patients with diabetic retinopathy.

# CHAPTER 8:
# EMERGING THERAPIES
# AND RESEARCH
# DIRECTIONS

## Stem Cell Therapy in Diabetic Retinopathy: Current Status and Future Perspectives

Stem cell therapy holds significant promise as a novel approach for the treatment of diabetic retinopathy (DR), offering the potential to restore retinal structure and function, promote tissue regeneration, and preserve visual acuity in individuals with diabetes mellitus (DM). Over the past decade, considerable progress has been made in the development of stem cell-based therapies for retinal diseases, including DR, leveraging the regenerative capacity of stem cells to address retinal vascular dysfunction, neurodegeneration, and macular pathology associated with the disease. This section provides an overview of stem cell therapy in diabetic retinopathy, highlighting its current status, therapeutic applications, challenges, and future directions.

## Stem Cells and Retinal Regeneration:

1 **Types of Stem Cells:** Stem cells are undifferentiated cells capable of self-renewal and differentiation into specialized cell types, offering the potential to regenerate damaged tissues and organs in various disease conditions. Several types of stem cells have been investigated for their therapeutic potential in diabetic retinopathy, including embryonic stem cells (ESCs), induced pluripotent stem cells (iPSCs), mesenchymal stem cells (MSCs), and retinal progenitor cells (RPCs), each with unique properties and differentiation capacities suitable for retinal regeneration and repair.

2 **Regenerative Potential:** Stem cells have the ability to differentiate into retinal cell types, including photoreceptors, retinal pigment epithelial (RPE) cells, and retinal ganglion cells (RGCs), and integrate into the host retina, providing a source of new cells to replace damaged or dysfunctional retinal tissue in diabetic retinopathy. Additionally, stem cells secrete trophic factors, cytokines, and extracellular matrix components that promote retinal survival, angiogenesis, and neuroprotection, enhancing tissue repair mechanisms and supporting retinal function in diabetic eyes.

**Therapeutic Applications of Stem Cell Therapy:**

1 **Replacement Therapy:** Stem cell-based replacement therapy aims to replace damaged retinal cells with healthy, functional cells derived from stem cell sources, offering the potential to restore visual function and preserve retinal integrity in individuals with diabetic retinopathy. Transplanted stem cells can differentiate into photoreceptors, RPE cells, and other retinal cell types, integrating into the host retina and forming synaptic connections with existing neurons to enhance visual signal transmission and processing.

2 **Neuroprotection:** Stem cells exert neuroprotective effects on retinal neurons by secreting neurotrophic factors, anti-

inflammatory cytokines, and anti-apoptotic molecules that promote neuronal survival, axonal regeneration, and synaptic remodeling in diabetic retinopathy. Stem cell therapy can mitigate retinal neurodegeneration, preserve retinal function, and prevent progressive vision loss by modulating neuroinflammatory responses, oxidative stress, and excitotoxicity in the diabetic retina.

3 **Angiogenesis Modulation:** Stem cells possess angiogenic properties and can modulate retinal vascularization by promoting neovascular regression, stabilizing existing blood vessels, and inhibiting pathological angiogenesis in diabetic retinopathy. Stem cell-derived paracrine factors, such as vascular endothelial growth factor (VEGF), pigment epithelium-derived factor (PEDF), and angiopoietin-1 (Ang-1), regulate retinal vascular homeostasis, endothelial cell function, and pericyte recruitment, contributing to the normalization of retinal blood flow and permeability in diabetic eyes.

**Clinical Trials and Translational Challenges:**

1 **Clinical Trials:** Several clinical trials have been initiated to evaluate the safety, feasibility, and efficacy of stem cell therapy for diabetic retinopathy, including phase I/II trials assessing the use of ESC-derived retinal cells, iPSC-derived retinal cells, and MSC-based therapies in patients with advanced DR. Preliminary results from these trials have shown promising outcomes in terms of visual improvement, retinal structure restoration, and long-term safety of stem cell transplantation in diabetic eyes, although larger-scale studies are needed to validate these findings and establish the clinical utility of stem cell therapy in routine practice.

2 **Translational Challenges:** Despite the potential benefits of stem cell therapy, several translational challenges need to be addressed to facilitate its clinical translation and widespread adoption in the management of diabetic retinopathy. These

challenges include the optimization of cell manufacturing processes, standardization of cell characterization and quality control protocols, development of immunomodulatory strategies to prevent graft rejection, and establishment of long-term safety monitoring and post-transplantation follow-up protocols to assess the efficacy and durability of stem cell-based interventions in diabetic eyes.

## Future Directions and Considerations:

1 **Advanced Cell Therapies:** Emerging technologies, such as genome editing, tissue engineering, and three-dimensional (3D) organoid culture systems, hold promise for advancing stem cell-based therapies for diabetic retinopathy by enhancing cell engraftment, functionality, and integration into the host retina. Novel approaches, including the generation of retinal organoids from patient-derived iPSCs, offer personalized treatment options and disease modeling platforms for studying the pathogenesis of diabetic retinopathy and screening potential therapeutic interventions in vitro.

2 **Combination Therapies:** Combining stem cell therapy with pharmacological agents, gene therapy, and tissue engineering approaches may enhance the therapeutic efficacy of stem cell-based interventions for diabetic retinopathy by targeting multiple pathological mechanisms underlying retinal vascular dysfunction, neurodegeneration, and macular edema associated with the disease. Synergistic interactions between stem cells and adjunctive therapies could maximize therapeutic outcomes, promote tissue regeneration, and improve long-term visual prognosis in individuals with diabetes mellitus.

## Conclusion:

Stem cell therapy holds great promise as a transformative approach for the treatment of diabetic retinopathy, offering the potential to restore retinal structure and function, promote tissue regeneration, and preserve visual acuity in individuals with diabetes mellitus. While significant progress has been made in preclinical and clinical studies of stem cell-based interventions for diabetic retinopathy, several translational challenges need to be addressed to facilitate their clinical translation and widespread adoption in routine practice. Through interdisciplinary collaboration among stem cell biologists, ophthalmologists, retina specialists, and diabetes care providers, stem cell therapy can revolutionize the management of diabetic retinopathy, offering personalized treatment options and innovative strategies to address the unmet needs of patients with diabetes mellitus. By harnessing the regenerative potential of stem cells, we can pave the way for a future where vision loss due to diabetic retinopathy becomes a preventable and treatable condition, ultimately improving the quality of life and visual outcomes for individuals affected by diabetes mellitus.

## Gene Therapy in Diabetic Retinopathy: Harnessing Genetic Approaches for Treatment

Gene therapy has emerged as a promising approach for the treatment of diabetic retinopathy (DR), offering the potential to address underlying genetic factors, modulate disease pathways, and restore retinal homeostasis in individuals with diabetes mellitus (DM). By targeting specific genes implicated in the pathogenesis of DR, gene therapy aims to correct genetic defects, regulate gene expression, and mitigate retinal vascular dysfunction, neurodegeneration, and macular pathology associated with the disease. This section provides an overview of gene therapy in diabetic retinopathy, highlighting its principles, therapeutic applications, challenges, and future directions.

### Principles of Gene Therapy:

1 **Gene Delivery:** Gene therapy involves the delivery of therapeutic genes, genetic material, or gene editing tools into target cells or tissues to modulate gene expression, correct genetic defects, and restore normal cellular function. Various gene delivery vectors, including viral vectors (e.g., adeno-associated virus, lentivirus) and non-viral vectors (e.g., liposomes, nanoparticles), are utilized to deliver therapeutic genes to the retina, allowing for precise targeting and efficient transduction of retinal cells in diabetic eyes.

2 **Gene Editing:** Gene editing technologies, such as CRISPR-Cas9, zinc finger nucleases (ZFNs), and transcription activator-like effector nucleases (TALENs), enable precise modification of the genome by introducing, removing, or modifying specific DNA sequences within the target gene. Gene editing holds promise for correcting disease-causing mutations, disrupting pathogenic gene expression, and modulating disease pathways implicated in diabetic retinopathy, offering potential therapeutic benefits for individuals with DM.

**Therapeutic Applications of Gene Therapy:**

1 **Angiogenesis Modulation:** Gene therapy can modulate retinal angiogenesis by targeting key angiogenic factors, such as vascular endothelial growth factor (VEGF), angiopoietin-2 (Ang-2), and insulin-like growth factor (IGF), involved in the pathogenesis of diabetic retinopathy. Gene therapy approaches, including anti-VEGF gene therapy, gene silencing of pro-angiogenic factors, and gene delivery of angiogenic inhibitors, aim to normalize retinal vascularization, inhibit pathological neovascularization, and improve retinal perfusion in diabetic eyes.

2 **Neuroprotection:** Gene therapy holds promise for neuroprotective strategies in diabetic retinopathy by targeting genes involved in retinal neurodegeneration, oxidative stress, and inflammatory responses. Gene therapy approaches, such as

delivery of neurotrophic factors (e.g., brain-derived neurotrophic factor, ciliary neurotrophic factor) and anti-inflammatory cytokines (e.g., interleukin-10), aim to promote neuronal survival, axonal regeneration, and synaptic remodeling in the diabetic retina, thereby preserving visual function and preventing vision loss.

3 **Macular Edema Management:** Gene therapy offers novel approaches for the management of diabetic macular edema (DME) by targeting genes involved in retinal vascular permeability, fluid homeostasis, and inflammation. Gene therapy approaches, including gene delivery of tight junction proteins (e.g., occludin, claudin-5), anti-inflammatory cytokines (e.g., interleukin-1 receptor antagonist), and aquaporin regulators, aim to restore blood-retinal barrier integrity, reduce macular edema, and improve visual acuity in individuals with DME.

## Clinical Trials and Translational Challenges:

1 **Clinical Trials:** Several clinical trials have been initiated to evaluate the safety, feasibility, and efficacy of gene therapy for diabetic retinopathy, including phase I/II trials assessing the use of gene-based interventions in patients with advanced DR and DME. Preliminary results from these trials have shown promising outcomes in terms of visual improvement, anatomical stabilization, and long-term safety of gene therapy approaches in diabetic eyes, although larger-scale studies are needed to validate these findings and establish the clinical utility of gene therapy in routine practice.

2 **Translational Challenges:** Despite the potential benefits of gene therapy, several translational challenges need to be addressed to facilitate its clinical translation and widespread adoption in the management of diabetic retinopathy. These challenges include optimizing gene delivery vectors for efficient transduction of retinal cells, minimizing off-target effects and immune responses, ensuring long-term expression and durability of therapeutic

genes, and developing personalized treatment strategies based on individual genetic profiles and disease characteristics.

### Future Directions and Considerations:

1 **Advanced Gene Editing Technologies:** Advances in gene editing technologies, such as base editing, prime editing, and epigenome editing, offer new opportunities for precise modification of the genome and targeted regulation of gene expression in diabetic retinopathy. These advanced gene editing tools enable site-specific correction of disease-causing mutations, modulation of gene expression levels, and epigenetic modifications to restore normal cellular function and mitigate disease progression in diabetic eyes.

2 **Combination Therapies:** Combining gene therapy with pharmacological agents, stem cell transplantation, and other therapeutic modalities may enhance the therapeutic efficacy of gene-based interventions for diabetic retinopathy by targeting multiple pathological mechanisms underlying retinal vascular dysfunction, neurodegeneration, and macular edema associated with the disease. Synergistic interactions between gene therapy and adjunctive therapies could maximize therapeutic outcomes, promote retinal regeneration, and improve long-term visual prognosis in individuals with diabetes mellitus.

### Conclusion:

Gene therapy represents a promising therapeutic approach for the treatment of diabetic retinopathy, offering the potential to modulate disease pathways, restore retinal homeostasis, and preserve visual function in individuals with diabetes mellitus. While significant progress has been made in preclinical and clinical studies of gene-based interventions for diabetic retinopathy, several translational challenges need to be addressed to facilitate their clinical translation and widespread adoption in routine practice. Through interdisciplinary collaboration among geneticists, ophthalmologists, retina specialists, and diabetes care providers, gene therapy can revolutionize the management of diabetic retinopathy, offering personalized treatment options and innovative strategies to address the unmet needs of patients with diabetes mellitus. By harnessing the power of gene editing and gene delivery technologies, we can pave the way for a future where gene therapy becomes a safe, effective, and transformative approach for the treatment of diabetic retinopathy, ultimately improving the quality of life and visual outcomes for individuals affected by diabetes mellitus.

## Neuroprotective Agents in Diabetic Retinopathy: Preserving Retinal Function and Structure

Neuroprotective agents have emerged as promising therapeutic strategies for the management of diabetic retinopathy (DR), focusing on preserving retinal function, promoting neuronal survival, and preventing neurodegeneration in individuals with diabetes mellitus (DM). By targeting key pathways involved in retinal neurodegeneration, oxidative stress, and inflammatory responses, neuroprotective agents aim to mitigate neuronal injury, enhance synaptic plasticity, and maintain visual function in diabetic eyes. This section provides an overview of neuroprotective agents in diabetic retinopathy, highlighting their mechanisms of action, therapeutic applications, challenges, and future directions.

### Mechanisms of Neurodegeneration in Diabetic Retinopathy:

1 **Retinal Neuronal Damage:** Diabetic retinopathy is characterized by progressive neuronal damage, including dysfunction and loss of retinal ganglion cells (RGCs), amacrine cells, bipolar cells, and photoreceptors, leading to impaired

visual function and vision loss in individuals with DM. Neurodegeneration in diabetic retinopathy is mediated by multiple pathogenic mechanisms, including oxidative stress, neuroinflammation, mitochondrial dysfunction, excitotoxicity, and vascular dysregulation, which contribute to synaptic dysfunction, axonal degeneration, and apoptotic cell death in the diabetic retina.

2 **Oxidative Stress:** Oxidative stress plays a central role in the pathogenesis of neurodegeneration in diabetic retinopathy, leading to the accumulation of reactive oxygen species (ROS), lipid peroxidation, protein oxidation, and DNA damage in retinal neurons. Increased oxidative stress disrupts cellular homeostasis, impairs mitochondrial function, and triggers apoptotic signaling pathways, contributing to neuronal injury, synaptic dysfunction, and retinal cell death in diabetic eyes.

3 **Inflammatory Responses:** Neuroinflammation is a key contributor to neuronal damage and degeneration in diabetic retinopathy, characterized by activation of microglia, infiltration of immune cells, and upregulation of pro-inflammatory cytokines, such as tumor necrosis factor-alpha (TNF-α), interleukin-1 beta (IL-1β), and interleukin-6 (IL-6), in the diabetic retina. Chronic inflammation exacerbates neuronal injury, disrupts synaptic connectivity, and impairs neurovascular coupling, leading to progressive neurodegeneration and vision loss in diabetic eyes.

**Neuroprotective Strategies in Diabetic Retinopathy:**

1 **Antioxidant Therapy:** Antioxidant agents, such as vitamins C and E, alpha-lipoic acid, coenzyme Q10, and N-acetylcysteine, exert neuroprotective effects by scavenging free radicals, reducing oxidative stress, and restoring redox balance in the diabetic retina. Antioxidants prevent neuronal damage, preserve mitochondrial function, and enhance neurotrophic support, promoting neuronal survival, synaptic plasticity, and visual function in

individuals with diabetic retinopathy.

2 **Anti-inflammatory Agents:** Anti-inflammatory agents, including corticosteroids, non-steroidal anti-inflammatory drugs (NSAIDs), and minocycline, mitigate neuroinflammation, suppress microglial activation, and inhibit pro-inflammatory cytokine production in the diabetic retina. Anti-inflammatory therapy attenuates neurodegeneration, preserves synaptic integrity, and improves retinal function by modulating neuroinflammatory responses and reducing neuronal injury in diabetic eyes.

3 **Neurotrophic Factors:** Neurotrophic factors, such as brain-derived neurotrophic factor (BDNF), nerve growth factor (NGF), and glial cell line-derived neurotrophic factor (GDNF), promote neuronal survival, stimulate axonal regeneration, and enhance synaptic connectivity in the diabetic retina. Neurotrophic factor therapy supports retinal neuroprotection, restores neurovascular interactions, and preserves visual function by promoting neuronal resilience and adaptive responses to metabolic stress in diabetic eyes.

## Clinical Trials and Translational Challenges:

1 **Clinical Trials:** Several clinical trials have investigated the efficacy of neuroprotective agents in diabetic retinopathy, including antioxidant supplements, anti-inflammatory medications, and neurotrophic factor therapies, in patients with mild to moderate DR and early diabetic macular edema (DME). Preliminary results from these trials have shown promising outcomes in terms of visual improvement, neuroprotection, and retinal structure preservation in diabetic eyes, although larger-scale studies are needed to confirm these findings and establish the clinical efficacy of neuroprotective agents in routine practice.

2 **Translational Challenges:** Despite the potential benefits of neuroprotective agents, several translational challenges need to

be addressed to facilitate their clinical translation and widespread adoption in the management of diabetic retinopathy. These challenges include optimizing drug delivery systems for efficient targeting of retinal neurons, minimizing systemic side effects and off-target effects, ensuring long-term safety and efficacy of neuroprotective agents, and developing personalized treatment strategies based on individual disease severity and progression in diabetic eyes.

## Future Directions and Considerations:

1 **Combination Therapies:** Combining neuroprotective agents with existing treatments, such as anti-VEGF therapy, laser photocoagulation, and pharmacological interventions, may enhance therapeutic efficacy and synergistically target multiple pathological mechanisms underlying diabetic retinopathy. Combination therapy approaches offer the potential to maximize neuroprotection, preserve retinal function, and improve visual outcomes in individuals with diabetes mellitus, particularly those with advanced DR and neurodegenerative changes in the retina.

2 **Precision Medicine:** Advancements in precision medicine, including biomarker discovery, genetic profiling, and molecular imaging techniques, may facilitate personalized treatment approaches tailored to individual patient characteristics and disease phenotypes in diabetic retinopathy. Precision medicine strategies enable early detection of neurodegenerative changes, identification of high-risk patients, and selection of optimal neuroprotective interventions based on genetic predisposition, disease severity, and treatment response in diabetic eyes.

## Conclusion:

Neuroprotective agents represent promising therapeutic strategies for the management of diabetic retinopathy, offering the potential to preserve retinal function, promote neuronal survival, and prevent neurodegeneration in individuals with diabetes mellitus. While significant progress has been made in preclinical and clinical studies of neuroprotective agents for diabetic retinopathy, several translational challenges need to be addressed to facilitate their clinical translation and widespread adoption in routine practice. Through interdisciplinary collaboration among neuroscientists, ophthalmologists, retina specialists, and diabetes care providers, neuroprotective agents can revolutionize the management of diabetic retinopathy, offering personalized treatment options and innovative strategies to address the unmet needs of patients with diabetes mellitus. By targeting neurodegenerative pathways and preserving retinal integrity, neuroprotective agents have the potential to improve visual outcomes and enhance quality of life for individuals affected by diabetic retinopathy.

# CHAPTER 9: HOLISTIC APPROACHES AND PATIENT EDUCATION

## Importance of Nutritional Counseling in Diabetic Retinopathy Management

Nutritional counseling plays a pivotal role in the comprehensive management of diabetic retinopathy (DR), offering personalized dietary guidance, lifestyle modifications, and nutritional interventions to optimize ocular health, prevent disease progression, and improve visual outcomes in individuals with diabetes mellitus (DM). By addressing dietary factors, nutrient deficiencies, and metabolic imbalances associated with diabetes, nutritional counseling aims to promote retinal health, mitigate vascular dysfunction, and support holistic well-being in diabetic patients. This section highlights the importance of nutritional counseling in DR management, emphasizing its role in disease prevention, glycemic control, and ocular health promotion.

### Disease Prevention and Risk Reduction:

1 **Dietary Patterns:** Nutritional counseling empowers individuals with diabetes to adopt healthy dietary patterns, such as the

Mediterranean diet, Dietary Approaches to Stop Hypertension (DASH) diet, and plant-based eating, which have been associated with reduced risk of diabetic retinopathy development and progression. These dietary patterns emphasize the consumption of nutrient-rich foods, including fruits, vegetables, whole grains, lean proteins, and healthy fats, while limiting intake of processed foods, sugary beverages, and high-glycemic index carbohydrates, which can exacerbate metabolic dysfunction and vascular damage in the retina.

2 **Weight Management:** Nutritional counseling promotes weight management and obesity prevention, addressing modifiable risk factors for diabetic retinopathy, such as central adiposity, insulin resistance, and dyslipidemia. By incorporating portion control, calorie moderation, and mindful eating practices, nutritional counseling helps individuals achieve and maintain a healthy body weight, reduce adipose tissue inflammation, and improve insulin sensitivity, thereby lowering the risk of developing diabetic retinopathy and other microvascular complications associated with obesity and metabolic syndrome.

**Glycemic Control and Metabolic Regulation:**

1 **Carbohydrate Management:** Nutritional counseling educates patients with diabetes about carbohydrate counting, meal timing, and glycemic index/load considerations to optimize blood glucose control and minimize postprandial hyperglycemia, which can contribute to retinal vascular dysfunction and oxidative stress. By balancing carbohydrate intake with insulin or oral glucose-lowering medications, nutritional counseling helps stabilize blood sugar levels, reduce glycemic variability, and prevent glucose-induced damage to retinal endothelial cells and pericytes, thereby preserving retinal microvascular integrity and function.

2 **Macronutrient Balance:** Nutritional counseling emphasizes the importance of balanced macronutrient intake, including carbohydrates, proteins, and fats, in maintaining metabolic

homeostasis and supporting ocular health in individuals with diabetes. By promoting a well-rounded diet that incorporates complex carbohydrates, lean proteins, and heart-healthy fats, nutritional counseling helps regulate blood lipids, reduce systemic inflammation, and optimize cellular metabolism, which are critical for preventing microvascular complications, including diabetic retinopathy.

**Ocular Nutrition and Antioxidant Supplementation:**

1 **Nutrient-Rich Foods:** Nutritional counseling encourages the consumption of nutrient-rich foods that support ocular health and provide essential vitamins, minerals, and antioxidants implicated in the prevention and management of diabetic retinopathy. These include dark leafy greens (e.g., spinach, kale), colorful fruits and vegetables (e.g., berries, carrots), fatty fish (e.g., salmon, mackerel), nuts and seeds (e.g., almonds, flaxseeds), and whole grains, which are rich in lutein, zeaxanthin, omega-3 fatty acids, vitamins C and E, and zinc, known for their antioxidant and anti-inflammatory properties.

2 **Supplemental Therapy:** In addition to dietary interventions, nutritional counseling may include recommendations for antioxidant supplementation, such as vitamins C and E, lutein, zeaxanthin, and omega-3 fatty acids, which have been shown to reduce oxidative stress, improve retinal microcirculation, and enhance visual function in individuals with diabetic retinopathy. While supplementation should be tailored to individual needs and medical history, nutritional counseling can help patients make informed decisions about the use of dietary supplements as adjunctive therapy for ocular health support.

**Lifestyle Modifications and Holistic Wellness:**

1 **Behavioral Change:** Nutritional counseling fosters behavioral change and sustainable lifestyle modifications that promote long-term adherence to healthy dietary habits, physical activity, and

self-care practices in individuals with diabetes. By providing education, guidance, and support, nutritional counseling empowers patients to make informed choices about food selection, meal planning, and lifestyle behaviors that positively impact metabolic control, vascular health, and ocular wellness, leading to improved outcomes and quality of life.

2 **Holistic Wellness:** Nutritional counseling integrates holistic wellness principles, including stress management, sleep hygiene, and social support, into the treatment plan for diabetic retinopathy, recognizing the interconnectedness of physical, emotional, and psychological factors in disease management and prevention. By addressing psychosocial factors that influence dietary behaviors and health outcomes, nutritional counseling promotes holistic well-being and resilience in individuals with diabetes, enhancing their ability to cope with the challenges of living with a chronic condition and maintaining optimal ocular health over the long term.

## Conclusion:

Nutritional counseling is an essential component of the multidisciplinary approach to diabetic retinopathy management, offering personalized dietary guidance, lifestyle modifications, and nutritional interventions to optimize metabolic control, prevent disease progression, and promote ocular health in individuals with diabetes mellitus. By addressing dietary factors, glycemic control, and antioxidant supplementation, nutritional counseling empowers patients to make informed choices about food selection, meal planning, and lifestyle behaviors that support retinal function, mitigate vascular dysfunction, and improve visual outcomes in diabetic eyes. Through collaborative efforts between nutritionists, ophthalmologists, endocrinologists, and diabetes care providers, nutritional counseling plays a critical role in the holistic management of diabetic retinopathy, fostering behavioral change, promoting holistic wellness, and enhancing quality of life for individuals affected by diabetes mellitus. By incorporating nutritional counseling into routine diabetes care, we can empower patients to take control of their health, prevent complications, and achieve optimal ocular outcomes, ultimately improving their overall well-being and quality of life.

## Exercise and Physical Activity Recommendations for Diabetic Retinopathy Management

Exercise and physical activity play a crucial role in the management of diabetic retinopathy (DR), offering numerous benefits for retinal health, vascular function, glycemic control, and overall well-being in individuals with diabetes mellitus (DM). By incorporating regular exercise into their lifestyle, patients with DR can improve blood circulation, reduce inflammation, enhance antioxidant defenses, and mitigate the progression of retinal complications associated with diabetes. This section provides evidence-based recommendations for exercise and physical activity in DR management, highlighting their effects on ocular health, metabolic control, and systemic wellness.

### Benefits of Exercise for Diabetic Retinopathy:

1 **Improved Retinal Blood Flow:** Exercise increases retinal perfusion and blood flow, promoting vascular health and oxygen delivery to the retina, which is essential for maintaining retinal function and preventing ischemic damage in individuals with DR. Regular physical activity enhances microvascular circulation, reduces capillary dropout, and improves tissue oxygenation in the diabetic retina, leading to reduced risk of retinal ischemia, macular edema, and neovascularization.

2 **Reduced Oxidative Stress:** Exercise enhances antioxidant defenses and reduces oxidative stress in the diabetic retina,

counteracting the detrimental effects of free radicals and reactive oxygen species (ROS) on retinal cells and blood vessels. Physical activity upregulates endogenous antioxidant enzymes, such as superoxide dismutase (SOD) and catalase, while decreasing lipid peroxidation and protein oxidation in the diabetic retina, thereby protecting against oxidative damage and preserving retinal integrity.

3 **Enhanced Glycemic Control:** Exercise improves insulin sensitivity, glucose uptake, and glycemic control in individuals with diabetes, leading to reduced hyperglycemia, insulin resistance, and systemic inflammation, all of which contribute to the pathogenesis of DR. Regular physical activity lowers fasting blood glucose levels, postprandial glucose excursions, and HbA1c levels in diabetic patients, resulting in decreased risk of retinal microvascular complications and diabetic macular edema.

4 **Weight Management:** Exercise promotes weight loss, body composition improvement, and metabolic regulation in individuals with diabetes, addressing modifiable risk factors for DR development and progression, such as obesity, dyslipidemia, and hypertension. Regular physical activity reduces visceral adiposity, adipose tissue inflammation, and adipokine dysregulation, which are implicated in the pathogenesis of DR and other diabetic complications, thereby lowering the risk of vision-threatening retinal disorders.

**Exercise Recommendations for Diabetic Retinopathy:**

1 **Aerobic Exercise:** Engage in moderate-intensity aerobic exercise, such as brisk walking, cycling, swimming, or jogging, for at least 150 minutes per week, spread over 3-5 days, to improve cardiovascular fitness, metabolic health, and retinal circulation in individuals with DR. Aim for a target heart rate of 50-70% of maximum heart rate during aerobic exercise sessions, gradually increasing duration, intensity, and frequency as tolerated.

2 **Resistance Training:** Incorporate resistance training or strength exercises, such as weightlifting, resistance band exercises, or bodyweight exercises, into your exercise routine at least 2 days per week, targeting major muscle groups and performing 8-12 repetitions per set. Resistance training improves muscle strength, bone density, and insulin sensitivity, supporting glycemic control and metabolic health in diabetic patients, while reducing the risk of falls and musculoskeletal injuries.

3 **Flexibility and Balance Exercises:** Include flexibility and balance exercises, such as yoga, tai chi, Pilates, or stretching routines, to enhance joint mobility, flexibility, and proprioception, reducing the risk of musculoskeletal injuries and improving functional capacity in individuals with DR. Incorporate gentle stretching exercises and balance drills into your daily routine to improve posture, coordination, and stability, which are important for maintaining mobility and preventing falls in diabetic patients.

**Precautions and Considerations:**

1 **Consultation with Healthcare Provider:** Before starting any exercise program, consult with your healthcare provider, ophthalmologist, or diabetes care team to assess your individual health status, vision impairment, and risk factors for exercise-related complications in diabetic retinopathy. Discuss any pre-existing eye conditions, retinal abnormalities, or vision changes that may affect your ability to engage in certain types of physical activity and receive personalized recommendations tailored to your needs and preferences.

2 **Eye Protection:** Wear appropriate eye protection, such as sunglasses with UV protection and sports goggles, when engaging in outdoor activities or high-risk sports to prevent eye injuries, phototoxicity, and exacerbation of retinal damage in individuals with DR. Choose sunglasses with polarized lenses and wrap-

around frames to minimize glare, enhance contrast sensitivity, and protect against ultraviolet (UV) radiation exposure, which can exacerbate retinal inflammation and oxidative stress in diabetic eyes.

3 **Monitoring for Symptoms:** Monitor for signs and symptoms of retinal complications, such as vision changes, floaters, flashes of light, or peripheral vision loss, during and after exercise sessions, and seek immediate medical attention if you experience any sudden onset or worsening of visual symptoms suggestive of retinal detachment, vitreous hemorrhage, or neovascularization in diabetic retinopathy. Be vigilant for warning signs of hypoglycemia, hyperglycemia, or cardiovascular events during exercise, and take appropriate measures to maintain safety and well-being.

**Gradual Progression and Individualization:**

1 **Gradual Progression:** Gradually increase the duration, intensity, and frequency of exercise sessions over time, starting with low-impact activities and progressing to moderate-intensity or vigorous exercises as tolerated and recommended by your healthcare provider. Avoid sudden increases in exercise volume or intensity, which may increase the risk of injury, exacerbate retinal complications, or trigger acute metabolic fluctuations in diabetic patients with DR.

2 **Individualization:** Tailor your exercise program to your individual preferences, capabilities, and health status, considering factors such as age, fitness level, mobility limitations, comorbidities, and visual impairment associated with diabetic retinopathy. Choose activities that you enjoy and can sustain long term, whether it's walking, cycling, swimming, dancing, or participating in group fitness classes, and modify exercises as needed to accommodate any vision-related challenges or safety concerns.

## Conclusion:

Exercise and physical activity are integral components of diabetic retinopathy management, offering numerous benefits for retinal health, metabolic control, and overall well-being in individuals with diabetes mellitus. By incorporating regular aerobic exercise, resistance training, flexibility exercises, and balance drills into their lifestyle, patients with DR can improve blood circulation, reduce oxidative stress, enhance glycemic control, and mitigate the progression of retinal complications associated with diabetes. Through collaborative efforts between healthcare providers, ophthalmologists, and diabetes educators, exercise recommendations can be tailored to individual needs, preferences, and health status, empowering patients to take control of their ocular health, prevent vision loss, and achieve optimal outcomes in diabetic retinopathy management. By embracing a physically active lifestyle, individuals with diabetes can enhance their quality of life, reduce their risk of diabetic complications, and enjoy the benefits of improved retinal function and visual well-being for years to come.

## Psychosocial Support for Patients with Diabetic Retinopathy: Enhancing Well-being and Coping Strategies

Psychosocial support plays a crucial role in the holistic management of diabetic retinopathy (DR), offering emotional, social, and psychological assistance to individuals coping with the challenges of living with vision loss and managing a chronic disease like diabetes mellitus (DM). By addressing the psychosocial impact of DR, healthcare providers can help patients navigate the emotional distress, functional limitations, and lifestyle adjustments associated with vision impairment, empowering them to maintain resilience, adaptability, and quality of life amidst the complexities of their condition. This section explores the importance of psychosocial support for patients with DR and provides strategies for enhancing well-being and coping.

## Understanding the Psychosocial Impact of Diabetic Retinopathy:

1 **Emotional Distress:** Diabetic retinopathy can evoke a range of emotional responses, including fear, anxiety, depression, frustration, and grief, as individuals grapple with the uncertainty, loss of independence, and perceived threat to their vision and quality of life. Vision loss can significantly impact self-esteem, self-efficacy, and mental well-being, leading to feelings of isolation, social withdrawal, and psychological distress in patients with DR.

2 **Functional Limitations:** Vision impairment can impose functional limitations on daily activities, such as reading, driving, cooking, and mobility, affecting individuals' autonomy, productivity, and sense of competence in managing their daily lives. Functional challenges associated with DR may require adaptations, assistive devices, and environmental modifications to facilitate independent living and maintain functional autonomy despite vision loss.

3 **Social Isolation:** Vision loss can contribute to social isolation, reduced social participation, and diminished quality of relationships, as individuals with DR may experience barriers to communication, transportation, and community engagement due to their visual impairment. Social isolation can exacerbate feelings of loneliness, alienation, and psychological distress, further compromising patients' mental health and well-being in the context of chronic illness.

## Strategies for Psychosocial Support:

1 **Education and Counseling:** Provide education and counseling to patients with DR about the psychosocial impact of vision loss, coping strategies, and resources available for emotional support, such as support groups, counseling services, and peer mentorship programs. Empower patients to express their concerns, fears, and emotional reactions to vision loss, validating their experiences and offering empathetic listening and emotional support.

2 **Peer Support Networks:** Facilitate connections with peer support networks, advocacy organizations, and community resources for individuals with DR, allowing patients to connect with others who share similar experiences, challenges, and coping strategies related to vision loss and diabetes management. Peer support networks provide emotional validation, practical guidance, and social connection, fostering a sense of belonging, empowerment, and resilience in patients facing similar health challenges.

3 **Cognitive-Behavioral Interventions:** Offer cognitive-behavioral interventions, such as relaxation techniques, mindfulness meditation, and stress management strategies, to help patients cope with anxiety, depression, and emotional distress associated with DR and vision loss. Teach patients adaptive coping skills, problem-solving strategies, and cognitive restructuring techniques to reframe negative thoughts, enhance resilience, and improve emotional well-being amidst the challenges of living with chronic illness.

**Rehabilitation Services:**

1 **Low Vision Rehabilitation:** Refer patients with DR to low vision rehabilitation services, including orientation and mobility training, vision rehabilitation therapy, and assistive technology assessments, to help them optimize their remaining vision, adapt to functional challenges, and maintain independence in daily activities. Low vision rehabilitation professionals can assess

patients' visual functioning, prescribe appropriate visual aids, and teach adaptive strategies for maximizing functional vision and quality of life despite vision loss.

2 **Occupational Therapy:** Involve occupational therapists in the care of patients with DR to address functional limitations, environmental barriers, and activities of daily living (ADL) challenges associated with vision impairment. Occupational therapists can provide training in adaptive techniques, home modifications, and assistive devices to enhance patients' independence, safety, and participation in meaningful activities, such as cooking, grooming, and leisure pursuits, despite visual limitations.

### Family and Caregiver Support:

1 **Family Education:** Educate family members and caregivers about the psychosocial impact of DR, vision loss, and diabetes management on patients' emotional well-being, functional independence, and quality of life. Encourage open communication, empathy, and support within the family unit, fostering a supportive environment that acknowledges patients' needs, concerns, and preferences in coping with chronic illness and vision impairment.

2 **Caregiver Support:** Provide support and resources for caregivers of individuals with DR, recognizing the challenges and burdens associated with caring for a loved one with vision loss and chronic illness. Offer caregiver education, respite care services, and support groups to help caregivers manage their own stress, maintain their well-being, and cope with the demands of caregiving while supporting the needs of their loved ones with DR.

### Conclusion:

Psychosocial support is essential for promoting resilience, well-being, and adaptation in individuals with diabetic retinopathy, helping them navigate the emotional, social, and functional challenges associated with vision loss and chronic illness. By addressing the psychosocial impact of DR and providing strategies for coping, healthcare providers can empower patients to maintain emotional resilience, functional independence, and quality of life despite the complexities of their condition. Through a multidisciplinary approach that integrates education, counseling, rehabilitation services, and caregiver support, patients with DR can enhance their coping skills, social support networks, and overall well-being, fostering a sense of empowerment, connection, and resilience in the face of vision loss and chronic illness.

## Patient Education on Self-Monitoring and Early Warning Signs in Diabetic Retinopathy

Effective patient education on self-monitoring and early warning signs is crucial in the management of diabetic retinopathy (DR), empowering individuals with diabetes mellitus (DM) to take an active role in monitoring their ocular health, detecting changes in vision, and seeking timely intervention to prevent vision loss and mitigate the progression of retinal complications. By providing comprehensive education on self-monitoring techniques, risk factors, and warning signs of DR, healthcare providers can empower patients to recognize subtle changes in their vision, adhere to recommended screening guidelines, and engage in proactive measures to preserve their visual function and quality of life. This section outlines key components of patient education on self-monitoring and early warning signs in DR management, emphasizing the importance of regular eye examinations, self-awareness, and prompt intervention to optimize ocular outcomes.

## Understanding Diabetic Retinopathy:

1 **Pathophysiology:** Educate patients about the pathophysiology of diabetic retinopathy, emphasizing the progressive nature of the disease and the risk factors associated with its development and progression, such as prolonged hyperglycemia, hypertension, dyslipidemia, and duration of diabetes. Explain how chronic hyperglycemia leads to microvascular damage, retinal ischemia, and neurodegeneration, contributing to the development of retinopathy and vision-threatening complications over time.

2 **Risk Factors:** Discuss modifiable and non-modifiable risk factors for diabetic retinopathy, including glycemic control, blood pressure management, lipid levels, smoking status, duration of diabetes, genetic predisposition, and comorbidities such as nephropathy and neuropathy. Encourage patients to address modifiable risk factors through lifestyle modifications, medication adherence, and regular healthcare visits to minimize the risk of retinal complications and optimize ocular outcomes.

## Importance of Regular Eye Examinations:

1 **Screening Guidelines:** Review recommended screening guidelines for diabetic retinopathy, emphasizing the importance of annual dilated eye examinations for individuals with diabetes, starting from the time of diagnosis for type 2 diabetes and within five years of diagnosis for type 1 diabetes. Explain that early detection and timely intervention are crucial for identifying retinal changes, monitoring disease progression, and implementing appropriate treatment strategies to prevent vision loss and preserve visual function.

2 **Comprehensive Eye Exams:** Educate patients about the components of a comprehensive eye examination for diabetic retinopathy, which includes dilated fundus examination, visual acuity assessment, intraocular pressure measurement, and

imaging modalities such as optical coherence tomography (OCT) and fluorescein angiography (FA) to evaluate retinal morphology and vascular leakage. Stress the importance of regular follow-up visits with an ophthalmologist or retina specialist to monitor changes in retinal health and adjust treatment plans as needed.

### Self-Monitoring Techniques:

1 **Visual Symptoms:** Teach patients to recognize common visual symptoms and warning signs of diabetic retinopathy, such as blurred vision, fluctuating vision, floaters, flashes of light, visual field defects, and sudden vision loss. Encourage patients to promptly report any changes in their vision to their healthcare provider, as these may indicate retinal complications requiring urgent evaluation and intervention to prevent irreversible vision loss.

2 **Home Monitoring:** Discuss self-monitoring techniques that patients can perform at home to assess their visual function and detect changes in vision between regular eye examinations. Encourage patients to use an Amsler grid or home vision testing kit to monitor for distortions, changes in central vision, or other abnormalities indicative of macular edema or macular degeneration. Emphasize the importance of regular self-assessment and timely reporting of any new or worsening visual symptoms to their healthcare provider.

### Adherence to Treatment and Lifestyle Modifications:

1 **Medication Adherence:** Stress the importance of medication adherence for managing diabetes and associated comorbidities, such as hypertension and dyslipidemia, to optimize glycemic control, blood pressure regulation, and lipid management, which are critical for preventing retinal complications and preserving visual function in diabetic patients.

2 **Lifestyle Modifications:** Encourage patients to adopt healthy

lifestyle habits, including maintaining a balanced diet, engaging in regular physical activity, quitting smoking, and managing stress, to promote overall health and reduce the risk of diabetic retinopathy progression. Provide guidance on dietary strategies for blood sugar control, such as carbohydrate counting, portion control, and glycemic index awareness, and emphasize the role of regular exercise in improving insulin sensitivity, cardiovascular fitness, and ocular circulation in individuals with diabetes.

## Collaboration and Follow-Up:

1 **Healthcare Team Collaboration:** Emphasize the importance of collaborative care between patients, primary care providers, endocrinologists, ophthalmologists, optometrists, and other members of the healthcare team in managing diabetic retinopathy and coordinating comprehensive diabetes care. Encourage patients to actively participate in their healthcare decisions, ask questions, and seek clarification on treatment recommendations and follow-up plans to ensure continuity of care and optimal ocular outcomes.

2 **Regular Follow-Up:** Reinforce the need for regular follow-up visits with healthcare providers, including ophthalmologists or retina specialists, to monitor retinal health, assess treatment efficacy, and adjust management strategies based on disease progression and individual patient response. Provide patients with a personalized follow-up schedule based on their risk profile, disease severity, and treatment regimen, ensuring timely intervention and proactive management of diabetic retinopathy to prevent vision loss and optimize visual outcomes over time.

## Conclusion:

Patient education on self-monitoring and early warning signs is essential in the management of diabetic retinopathy, empowering individuals with diabetes to recognize changes in their vision, adhere to recommended screening guidelines, and engage in proactive measures to preserve their ocular health and quality of life. By providing comprehensive education on diabetic retinopathy, screening recommendations, self-monitoring techniques, and lifestyle modifications, healthcare providers can empower patients to take an active role in managing their condition, preventing vision loss, and optimizing visual outcomes through regular eye examinations, medication adherence, and collaboration with the healthcare team. Through collaborative efforts between patients and healthcare providers, individuals with diabetic retinopathy can navigate the complexities of their condition, maintain resilience, and achieve optimal ocular health and well-being over the long term.

Printed in Great Britain
by Amazon